Tai Chi Ch'uan
THE CHINESE WAY

Tai Chi Ch'uan
THE CHINESE WAY

FOEN TJOENG LIE

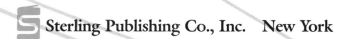
Sterling Publishing Co., Inc.   New York

Library of Congress Cataloging-in-Publication Data

Lie, Foen Tjoeng.
   [Chinesisches Schattenboxen Tai-Ji-Quan für geistige und
körperliche Harmonie. English]
   Tai chi ch'uan : the Chinese way / by Foen Tjoeng Lie ;
[translated by Elizabeth Reinersmann].
     p.   cm.
   Translation of: Chinesisches Schattenboxen Tai-Ji-Quan für
geistige und körperliche Harmonie.
   Includes index.
   ISBN 0-8069-6826-5 (pbk.)
   1. T'ai chi ch'üan.   I. Title.
GV504.L5413 1988   87-35928
613.7' 1—dc19   CIP

1   3   5   7   9   10   8   6   4   2

Translated by Elizabeth Reinersmann

Translation edited by Timothy Nolan

English translation copyright © 1988
by Sterling Publishing Co., Inc.
Two Park Avenue, New York, N.Y. 10016
Original edition published under the title "Chinesisches
Schattenboxen: Tai-Ji-Quan für geistige und körperliche
Harmonie" © 1987 Falken-Verlag Gmbh,
6272 Niedernhausen/Ts., West Germany
Distributed in Canada by Oak Tree Press Ltd.
% Canadian Manda Group, P.O. Box 920, Station U
Toronto, Ontario, Canada M8Z 5P9
Distributed in the United Kingdom by Blandford Press
Link House, West Street, Poole, Dorset BH15 1LL, England
Distributed in Australia by Capricorn Ltd.
P.O. Box 665, Lane Cove, NSW 2066
Manufactured in the United States of America
All rights reserved
Sterling ISBN 0-8069-6826-5 Paper

Photos: Studio Kade, Pressbaum (Austria)
Drawings: G. Scholz, Dornburg; Gabriele Hampel,
Kelkheim; Pia Seelback, Wiesbaden

Contents

The History and Effects of Tai Chi Ch'uan . . . *109*

Acknowledgments

I want to thank the many people who helped me, particularly Brigitte Brunner for her help in finishing the manuscript; Ilia Kaderavek for his tireless efforts and for the many helpful suggestions; Dr. Helga Berger and Dr. Michael Singer; and Gerhard Vasicek for the editing of the text. Their contributions made this book possible.

Preface

Tai chi ch'uan (Chinese shadowboxing) is an exercise of harmonious body movements. Chinese culture has always been concerned with the promotion of a well-functioning body, but recently the number of people in the West interested in tai chi ch'uan has gone up as well. Tai chi ch'uan increases awareness of the body and is an aid for meditation.

This book will not replace what a good teacher will teach you. But it will most certainly assist and guide you in understanding the basic features of the movements.

It is my hope that this book will convey to you the essence of tai chi ch'uan through the modified short form of 24 sequences, also known as the Peking form. It was introduced by the Sports Committee of the People's Republic of China and is the most popular form throughout the world. It is graceful and appealing while being easy to learn and master.

Introduction

Tai chi ch'uan is the name for a number of traditional Chinese exercises. Its characteristics are gentle movements that harmonize breathing with mental concentration against a particular philosophical background.

Tai chi, a concept in the philosophy of Taoism, refers to the condition of our Universe at the dawn of time. It is the source of heaven and earth, the Ying and the Yang. Ch'uan means the joy of fighting with bare fists; tai chi ch'uan as an exercise grew out of the Chinese art of fighting and many movements still show elements of self-defense.

Much emphasis in tai chi ch'uan is focused on the careful and flowing movements. The flow is gentle, harmonious, and graceful, which makes watching tai chi ch'uan an aesthetic experience. While the upper body remains nimble and loose, the lower part of the body and legs are stable and planted firmly on the ground without being stiff. Thus, tai chi ch'uan is one of the best forms of physical training. With consistent use, prevention and treatment of illness is possible.

The important principles of tai chi ch'uan are:
- Overcome force and severity with softness, gentleness, and smoothness.
- Move a ton with an ounce.
- Adapt your opponent's style, and beat him at it.

As a rule, all movements are performed in an archlike, rounded fashion, conforming to the Ying-Yang philosophy expressed in the tai chi symbol (Illus. 1).

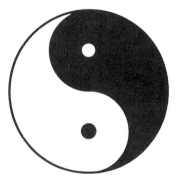

Illus. 1

The
Basics of
Tai Chi Ch'uan

Characteristics of Tai Chi Ch'uan

Tai chi ch'uan requires that your posture be steady and relaxed and your movements be harmonious, similar to the way the body operates. After a couple of rounds you will notice very little overexertion or shortness of breath. On the contrary, one should feel a physical and emotional exhilaration. This is why tai chi ch'uan is an ideal conditioning program.

Relaxation and Harmony

Tai chi ch'uan sequences should flow continuously without a break, even when you change positions or shift your weight. When you do tai chi ch'uan correctly the movements follow each other harmoniously and should look like floating clouds or flowing waters.

Flowing Motion

In contrast to other martial arts, tai chi ch'uan's movements are round, or arched, rather than straight. This makes for less stress, since round movements follow the natural motion of the body's joints.

Round and Natural Movements

The tai chi ch'uan movements have to be performed continuously, whether you choose the complete form or only a portion.

Coordinate the movements of the arms with those of the legs. Arm and leg movements originate from the torso; so synchronize them with each other. Let your mental control, depth of breathing, and body movements form a unit.

Coordination of the Whole Body

Criteria for the Exercises

Use the following criteria when doing the exercises. They will help you meet the characteristics of tai chi ch'uan just outlined.

Consciousness should guide all body movements (except reflective reactions) when doing tai chi ch'uan. In

Deliberate Control

addition to this emphasis on concentration, it is vital that you bring imagination to the process.

Here is an example: When you do the first sequence of the Peking form (p. 29) you will begin with a slow lifting of both arms forward to shoulder level. Rather than simply moving your arms upwards, visualize the movement first and then, slowly and relaxed, follow through.

Visualize all the movements in this way before actually doing them. You can't do tai chi ch'uan correctly if you don't visualize first.

Here are two sayings that underline this thought: "Your mind guides your body," and "Your body will follow your thoughts." In order to fulfil these requirements, follow these other steps:

Calmness and Alertness

A calm but alert disposition is important when assuming the starting position. Do not allow your thoughts to ramble around. Clear your mind; then check the following:

- Is the position of your head and torso correct?
- Are your shoulders and arms relaxed?
- Are you breathing freely and easily?

Only when these preconditions are met should you proceed calmly with performing the movements.

Quiet is essential when concentrating on the individual movements with deliberate detail. If quiet is not observed, the danger of doing the exercises incorrectly or in the wrong order is very great.

The sayings are: "Quietness is the guide of movements," and "Through action calmness is maintained."

Form a mental picture and then practise with complete concentration. Remember, don't let your thoughts wander. It'll be difficult at first to remember this. But it is easy to pay too much attention to the individual movements and their coordination, and this will interfere with concentrating on the whole, which is essential. Over time and with enough patience you will perform your movements in a conscious response to a mental image, and these processes will be in full harmony with each other. This is your goal.

During tai chi ch'uan you are in a relaxed (not lax or limp) state. Your muscles and joints are not tense and the body is able to work on particular positions. The movements are not stiff, heavy, or abrupt. The spine is in a natural erect position and should not be overly extended. The head, torso, arms, and legs should be able to move freely and gently. The upper body is comfortably straight, never bending forward or backwards or leaning left or right. *Use only as much energy as is required for your body to achieve a certain position.* The Chinese word for this is *jing* ("real energy" or "inner energy"). Use only your jing for arm and leg movements and keep the rest of the body as relaxed as possible.

It is not easy in the beginning to determine the proper amount of jing energy. In order to learn how to apply the proper amount of energy it is recommended that, first, limber up your body and pay attention to how much energy you use. In this way arms and legs can move more freely and you can perform all your movements with as little energy as possible. Once you have done this all your movements will be gentle and have the desired roundness. They will flow into each other and will be coordinated.

Relaxing versus Energy Expending

Since your mental visualizations guide your body movements, tai chi ch'uan is a training program for the whole person.

These coordinated, harmonious movements help to integrate the existing physical condition of a person with his or her potential, leading to the improvement of the mind as well as the body. This, in turn, will influence the mood and add to a state of psychological balance. This is why tai chi ch'uan puts so much emphasis on coordination.

Coordination is a "dialogue of movements" expressed in these sayings: "If one part of the body is in motion, the rest cannot remain still," or "The whole of the body moves in one breath: from legs to spine to arms." Thus, the movement of one part (arms) should be in harmony with the movement of another part (legs). From the very beginning, attempt to make the spine or, better, the center of the abdomen (Dan-Tian, see p. 17), the center

Coordination

15

from which all movements start and from where they flow to the extremities.

In the beginning, try not to do the complete form all at once. Practise only a portion of it, for example, Sequence 1 (The Beginning) or Sequence 10 (Move Hands Like Clouds). Use these to practise the coordination of the extremities. From there move on to the "rider position" and "marksman position." Both are good to practise shifting your weight and changing your steps. The result will be a good command of the step sequences and a solid footing.

Go through each sequence one by one in order to synchronize the steps with the hand and body movements. From this you will achieve the greatest coordination of the body and better conditioning.

Weight Shifting and Center of Gravity

Even distribution of weight and solid footings are both important in tai chi ch'uan. Both play a key roll when you have to change a position; so there must not be any doubt which leg is carrying the greater portion of weight (in Chinese: *shi*= "fullness," or "full") and which leg carries only a minimum (in Chinese: *xue*= "emptiness," or "empty"). Shift in a flowing motion. When the distinction between "fullness" and "emptiness" is not clear, stable footing is not possible and the body posture will be shaky. Everything will look and feel awkward.

Tai chi ch'uan when describing the meaning of nimble and sure-footed steps and skilful and precise hand movement makes the following comparison: "Walk like a cat and move your hands as if pulling a silken thread."

Pay attention distributing and shifting your weight in order to maintain good balance and assure calm, even movements of your arms and legs. Without balance it is impossible to remain on solid footing, let alone to move with agility and precision.

No matter how difficult or complex a movement is, try first and most of all to achieve this state of steadiness combined with relaxation. The words that describe one of tai chi ch'uan's most important preconditions are: "Middle, upright, calm, and comfortable." For example:

- Stand erect on solid footing before you turn your body;
- Plant your feet solidly on the ground before you shift the center of gravity of your body.

Additional criteria for a stable center of gravity are:
- dropping shoulders;
- "letting go" of your spine and hips (see p. 20);
- deep breathing from the diaphragm.

When you pay attention to these criteria, calmness and agility will be your reward.

Tai chi ch'uan requires deep and calm breathing out of and into the center of the abdomen (Dan-Tian). Lower and raise the diaphragm with each breath as deliberately as possible without straining. Follow the technique of the "moving diaphragm" by consciously focusing on the process.

Natural Breathing

This is what tai chi ch'uan means by "guiding the Qi (breath) into the Dan-Tian." This type of deep breathing from the center of the abdomen stimulates not only the internal organs but also the nervous system. Over time one can notice a certain warm, comfortable "Qi-feeling" in the center of the abdomen.

Breathing is innately coordinated with the movements of the body. For example, you exhale when you get up and inhale when you sit down; you exhale when you stretch your arms and inhale when you fold them. Make sure that breathing remains calm and natural, never forced or slowed down. If you are not familiar with the Qi/Dan-Tian breathing technique, try in the beginning to concentrate on normal and quiet breathing. Breathe as you have done all along. The body is capable, intuitively, of regulating the breathing process according to a given situation.

In the beginning pay attention only to your normal breathing. Wait until you are familiar with the movements of the form, and then begin to tackle the new breathing process (unless, of course, you are already familiar with that technique). The coordination between movements and breathing should never be forced or mechanical. Rather, in tai chi ch'uan the amount of breathing is determined by the physiological needs of each individual as well as personal experiences, abilities and conditioning.

There may be a need to adjust your breathing when doing an individual movement. This is a physical need, and if not met can cause disharmony, shortness of breath, pain, or rapid pulse. At the very least it will create disharmony in the movement itself.

All the criteria listed above represent a unified whole. For example: If you are tense you will not be able to concentrate; consequently, you will not be able to mentally visualize and guide the process, resulting in movements that are not round and flowing. Shifting your weight from one foot to another will not be done properly and balance will be lost. That, in turn, will result in a tensing up which will interfere with the process of coordination and, finally, will affect proper and natural breathing.

Instructions for Body Posture

Head

In tai chi ch'uan the head is in a natural erect position. This is very important, since the head, torso, and spine form a unit. Consequently, the position of the head influences the posture of the body.

In order to keep the head in the desired position, the neck muscles must remain relaxed without letting the head bob about, lean to either side, or fall forward or back. Try to picture having something on your head that you are trying to push up. Do this by using jing energy, just enough to get your head into the right position (see p. 15). Tai chi ch'uan calls this: "suspending the head" or "carrying the crown of the head high."

Move your head in unison with your body when you change direction or position, and when turning. Your facial muscles should always be relaxed and natural, the chin slightly pulled in, lips together (without effort), teeth slightly in contact, and the top of your tongue lightly touching a place directly behind your upper front teeth (again, without effort).

At the beginning of each sequence look peacefully forward. Do not stare or look bored, but be aware of the environment without being preoccupied with it. In this way your eyes will be able to follow the movements of your hands as well as the changing positions of your body. Look straight ahead at the end of the sequence.

Your audio senses should also be aware of the environment, again without being distracted, so that you can focus all attention on the exercises with a calm and relaxed disposition.

Chest and Back

In tai chi ch'uan your back is in a natural upright position. Relax your chest, without pulling in or pushing out, and stand normal and erect. This is essential for the correct breathing technique and is also important to avoid tension in the shoulders.

Allow your chest to expand and your diaphragm to move freely up and down. Let both shoulders hang down so that they can move freely in any direction. Tai chi ch'uan calls this, "holding back chest and pulling back straight." In this case, "holding back" does not mean pulling your chest inward. The Chinese word for this is *han*, and its meaning is best described by a comparison with a flower bud that is in the process of opening up. The chest is held back but ready at a moment's notice to "unfold." It is important for your chest to remain in this state throughout the tai chi ch'uan exercises.

Spine, Abdomen, and Hips

Your spinal column is always in control of your body, whether you are walking, standing, sitting, or lying down. The saying is, "The spinal column is the ruler of the body," or "The spiral column is the central axis for the body's movements." This is why a correct posture is so important, since it makes it possible to do exercises in comfort and with steadiness while being relaxed at the same time.

Keep the spinal column deliberately relaxed so that all movements are free of all tension, whether you move forward or backwards, turn, or shift your weight. This also guarantees that the center of gravity remains in balance which in turn assures that leg movements are steady, rounded and surefooted. All this is possible only if the spinal column, from the chest vertebrae on down, forms a straight vertical line. Now all tai chi ch'uan movements can be flawlessly performed, and the body posture will always be natural, upright, and correct.

Keep the muscles of the abdomen relaxed so that the breathing technique (that imaginary sinking down of the Qi to the center of the abdomen, the Dan-Tian) can be observed at all times. The Dan-Tian is three finger widths below the navel. Again, do all this with your jing. You want to be able to focus all your energy on the conscious awareness of your body.

Lower Body

In a normal position the buttock is pointing slightly backwards (Illus. 2 and 3). When you are standing it should "sink down" as if you where sitting on a stool or on a horse with a straight but relaxed back. This will keep the buttocks from sticking out too far (Illus. 4) which would bend the spinal column too far forward, causing the hips to stiffen and restricting movements to the legs.

You can do this by turning your pelvis slightly forward and up, hips relaxed. This will practically guarantee a vertical posture and will allow for an equal distribution of weight on the lower back, relieving the individual vertebrae (Illus. 5). Again, use jing energy to avoid tension and stiffness.

Legs and Feet

The stability of all tai chi ch'uan movements is in the legs. Therefore, pay special attention to all leg movements. Tai chi ch'uan says, "The forms are rooted in the feet, spring forth from the legs, get guidance from the pelvis, and find expression in the movements of the hands." This means that the position of the legs will determine the form and expression of a tai chi ch'uan exercise.

Your hips and knees should be relaxed but stable to avoid wobbly legs. When these joints are able to move freely and are relaxed, skilful, gentle and surefooted legwork is possible.

Your feet should move quickly and easily; when they move forward, the heel touches the floor first, when they move backwards the toes touch first. In the beginning it'll seem impossible to move your legs and arms

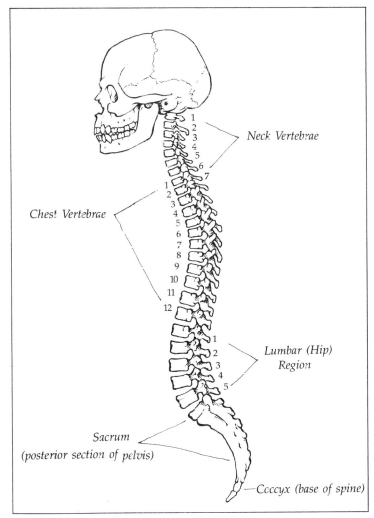

Neck Vertebrae

Chest Vertebrae

Lumbar (Hip)
Region

Sacrum
(posterior section of pelvis)

Coccyx (base of spine)

Illus. 2

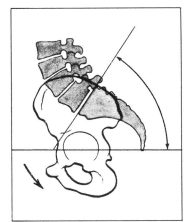

Illus. 3

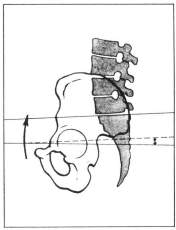

Illus. 4

Illus. 2. Normal position of spine

Illus. 3. Normal position of hip
and buttock

Illus. 4. Incorrect position of hip
and buttock. Note the stress on
the vertebrae

Illus. 5. Correct position for tai
chi ch'uan, with less stress on
vertebrae

Illus. 5

at the same time, and you'll want to neglect your legs in favor of your hands. But this will surely ruin the form. Try to move arms and legs simultaneously, and if it's too difficult at first, practice leg and arm movements separately, leg movements first. Concentrate on the positions and steps and make sure you understand the important leg movements. Pay attention to the weight distribution between both legs, which is very important throughout all sequences of tai chi ch'uan. There are only three sequences ("Beginning," "Conclusion," and "Crossing Hands") where your weight distribution will be equal.

Never be in doubt which leg supports the full weight (fullness) and which one is only carrying a small amount (empty). The "empty foot" should carry 1/10 or 1/8 of your weight.

Shifting your weight from one foot to the other must be a distinct movement, but not clumsy or stiff. This assures not only stability of the body but agility during the changing of steps. Because your weight constantly shifts you won't get muscle cramps and you won't feel tired as fast. Every step during tai chi ch'uan should be calm and unhurried. But most of all, make sure your body is well in balance and that you are calm and thinking about every movement before actually doing it.

Upper Extremities

Tai chi ch'uan says, "Let shoulders hang down and keep elbows slightly bent but relaxed." All your joints should be limber so that your movements can be round and gentle. Since all your joints are part of one another, a relaxed shoulder means a relaxed elbow. Keep in mind that the shoulders are slightly back and pressed outward to avoid a "pulling up."

Keep your hands and wrists relaxed and able to move freely without becoming limp. Slope your hands downwards very slightly when you pull them towards your body. Let your hands "fall down" at the wrists with your fingers pointing slightly backwards when you push ahead. Hands and wrists should be limber, fingers natural. When you turn your hands, do it very calmly, evenly, and relaxed. Your fists should also be limber and not "white-knuckled." Shoulders, arms, and hands should move in unison. If you push your hands too far forward your arms will stretch too far. That makes it impossible for your shoulders and elbows to hang. Likewise, if the shoulder and elbow movement is too extensive your hands can't push out far enough.

Follow these instructions for correct hand and arm movement:
- move naturally and be limber
- make movements gentle and round
- move with ease (but not flighty)
- let movements be solid but not stiff.

Each hand creates, individually, an image, while together their movements flow in unison.

Important Instruction for Tai Chi Ch'uan Exercises

As I said in the Preface, this book is not intended to replace a course in tai chi ch'uan. If for some reason you cannot take part in classroom exercises you should work in a group. Not only can you learn from each other and tackle problems better, but you will also encourage each other to stay "on the ball" and discourage each other from throwing in the towel too quickly. Besides, it is more fun and sociable to exercise in a group.

In addition to body posture, breathing technique, deliberate control, coordination, etc., the following are additional criteria that should be taken into consideration.

Perseverance

As with most things, perseverance is essential for the tai chi ch'uan exercises. Try to practise every day to complement the class or group activity. Practise before or after work, either early in the morning or late in the afternoon. Find a quiet place with lots of fresh air (like a park, garden, lakeside, or a quiet room). Practise regularly, even after you've mastered the whole form. Remember, practise makes perfect.

Even if perfection is seldom achieved, regular exercise will raise the level of expertise. One precondition for tai chi ch'uan is that you execute the form correctly. How fast or how much you learn is not important. What is important is taking the time to learn the form step by step—like a baby learning to walk.

If you have a problem with a particular movement, step, or position, do not go on to something new. Practise until you are in command; then go on to the next exercise.

Even Tempo

Do tai chi ch'uan in an even, slow tempo so it'll be easier to learn the individual elements of the form. Get used to an even tempo from the beginning. With only a few exceptions, tai chi ch'uan should be done this way from the first to the last sequence.

With moderate speed the complete shortened version of the Peking form can be done in 5 to 6 minutes (7 to 9 minutes if you choose a somewhat slower speed).

Even Heights

The heights of the body during the exercises are determined by the knee bend in the very first sequence ("Beginning"). Try to hold this height throughout the exercise (except for Sequences 16 and 17). It is advisable for less conditioned people, as well as for beginners, to moderate the knee bend to avoid too much strain. Once stamina has increased through consistent training the knee bends can be adjusted.

Stress Load

Tai chi ch'uan does not demand a high load of physical strain. Nevertheless, since the arms and legs are always moving in a slightly bent position, this activity does carry its share of stress. The legs are most affected, particularly in the beginning. Shifting your weight may make your muscles sore but with regular practice (if need be with a shortened exercise period) your legs will become stronger and the soreness will go away. How long and how often you exercise is a matter of motivation, condition and routine but a normal, healthy person should be able to exercise several times a day for a half hour without any problems. Only older people and those with a weak physical condition should take their particular situation into account, because too much stress can result in dizziness, limpness, weakness, and heavy perspiration.

A sure sign of too much stress is a pulse rate that is 20 beats per minute higher than it was at the beginning. This can be the result of a wrong breathing technique or a higher than recommended speed. If this should happen, reduce the amount and time of exercise. If need be, shorten the number of sequences, and maybe reduce the degree of the knee bends. It is always better to work moderately but regularly.

Too much of even a good thing can do more harm than good. People with a chronic illness should check with their physician to find out if and how much stress their system can tolerate and if tai chi ch'uan is the proper exercise for them.

The Peking Form

The Peking form, or shortened version, of tai chi ch'uan was developed in 1956 by the Sports Committee of the People's Republic of China. The 24 sequences use many forms of tai chi and are arranged from easiest to hardest. This makes the Peking form easy to learn, to understand, and to master.

- When you read "simultaneously," or "at the same time," execute the movements in unison, regardless of the sequence of their presentation.
- Directions for each movement are always given from the point of the person who does the exercise. "Forward" means straight ahead, "back" means behind you, likewise "left" and "right."
- The use of "east," "west," "south," etc., is meant as an aid for orientation. Always start your exercise facing south.

■■■■■■■■■■■■■■■■■■ *Note*

Before you get started, take a good look at the diagram on pages 106–107. It will give you an overview of the total Peking form, and help the beginner with proper positioning and direction while learning the form. It will also help you if you are advanced and attempting to execute the whole form.

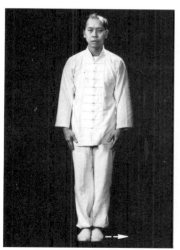 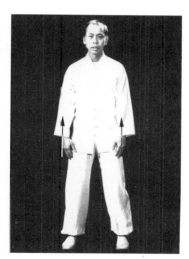

Illus. 6   *Illus. 7*

Sequence 1:
The Beginning
(Qi-Ji)

From a normal position, with your feet close together (Illus. 6), move them a shoulder's width apart. Stand

■■■■■■■■■■■■■■■■■■ *Step 1*

straight, with your knees relaxed, and your toes pointed forward. Keep your arms and hands loosely next to your body, palms turned towards your thighs. Look straight ahead (Illus. 7).

Note ▰▰▰▰▰▰▰▰▰ Keep your head and neck upright and pull your chin back very slightly. Do not move your chin forward, pull your stomach in, or pull your shoulders up. Keep your whole body relaxed and your mind alert, concentrating on the movements. Turn your toes inward slightly, so that you'll be ready for the next step. The distance between your heels should be about 12 inches.

Step 2 ▰▰▰▰▰▰▰▰▰ Move your hands up to shoulder level (Illus. 8, Illus. 9—side view), keeping your wrists relaxed and your arms straight. Your palms should face down (Illus. 10). Keep the distance between both hands a shoulder's width apart.

Step 3 ▰▰▰▰▰▰▰▰▰ Slowly bend your knees, keeping your upper body straight. This will create the "rider position." At the same time, let your hands "fall down" gently, as you push your wrists towards the floor. Bend your elbows until your lower arms are parallel to the floor: they should be in line with your knees, palms down. Look straight ahead.

Note ▰▰▰▰▰▰▰▰▰ Don't raise your shoulders as you move your arms up. Keep your elbows and wrists relaxed; fingers in their normal position. When you bend your knees, keep your spine and hips relaxed. Don't let your back and buttocks stick out. The center of gravity is between your legs, and your weight should be equally distributed between your right and left foot. Move your arms and legs in harmony.

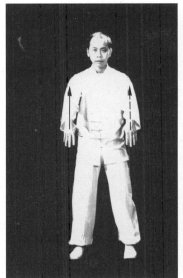

Illus. 8

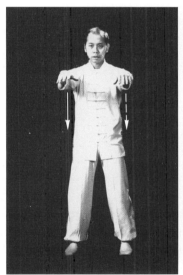

Illus. 9

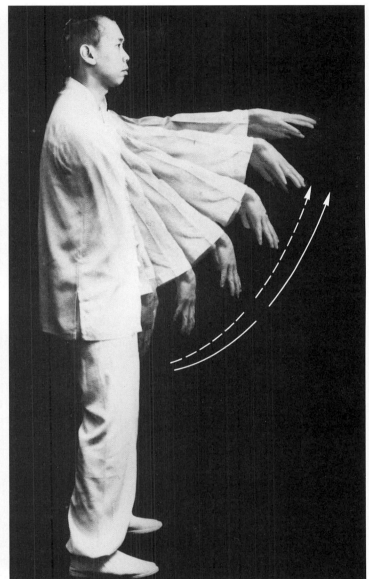

Illus. 10

Sequence 2: Parting a Wild Horse's Mane
(Zuo-You Ye-Ma Fen-Zong)

Step 1

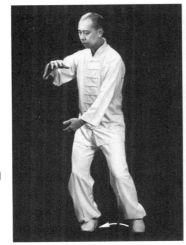

Illus. 12

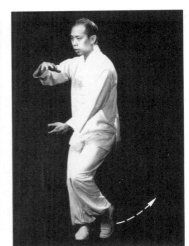

Illus. 13

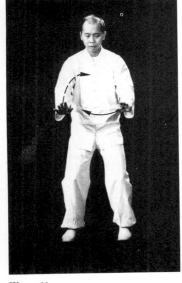

Illus. 11

Turn your body slightly to the right and shift your weight to your right foot. At the same time, move your right hand in an arch upwards to chest height and your left hand in an arch down in front of your stomach below your navel. Your palms should face each other; both elbows should "hang down" and bend (Illus. 12). This is called the "ball holding" position. Your left foot should rest next to your right but only the toe should touch the floor (Illus. 13).

Note

Don't bring your hands too close to your body. Otherwise, you have to bend your elbows too far and the position of your arms will not be "round" anymore.

Turn your body slightly to the left and push your left foot forward (Illus. 14). Move your left arm up and your right arm down until they are almost at the same level (Illus. 15). Lower your left foot to the floor, bending your knee slightly. Shift your weight to your left foot and continue to move your arms—your left one up and your right one down (Illus. 16).

Finish by relaxing and straightening your right leg; bringing your right hand, in an arch, straight down your side, palm down, and your left arm fully extended. Pull your palm back (Illus. 17). You are now in the "marksman position."

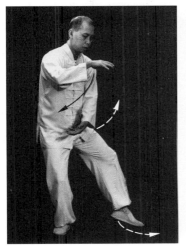

Illus. 14

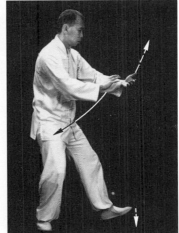

Illus. 15

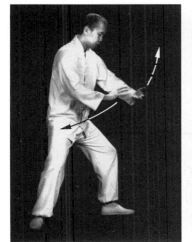

Illus. 16

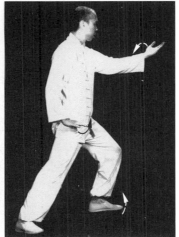

Illus. 17

Step 3 Shift your weight slowly back to your right foot as if you wanted to sit down. Raise your left foot up on its heel and turn on it 45° to the left before setting back on the floor. At the same time, move your left hand to chest height and turn your hand as if you wanted to cover up something. Move your right hand in an arch in front of your abdomen, and turn your hand as if you wanted to catch something. Your palms should face each other with both elbows relaxed and bent (Illus. 18). You are back in the ball holding position.

Now shift your weight back to your left foot and straighten your right, so your legs are in the marksman position (Illus. 19).

Pull your right foot up on its toes and bring it next to the left foot. Turn your body to the left until your left foot is supporting your total weight. Look at your left hand (Illus. 20).

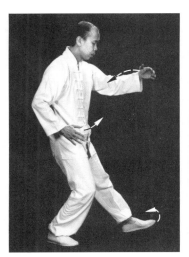

Illus. 18

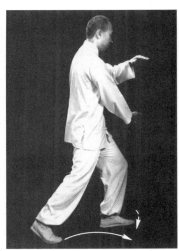

Illus. 19

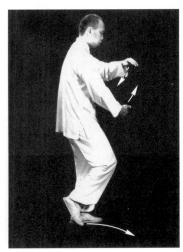

Illus. 20

Step 4 Turn your body to the right until it faces east. At the same time, move your right hand to eye level, your palm in front of your face on an angle (Illus. 21).

Simultaneously, step forward and right with your right foot, bend your right leg, and relax and straighten your left leg. This will shift your weight to your right foot and put you back in the marksman position (Illus. 22).

Now move your left hand, in an arch, to your hip, then down, with your palm facing the floor, fingertips forward (Illus. 23). Both elbows should be bent slightly. Look to your right hand (Illus. 24).

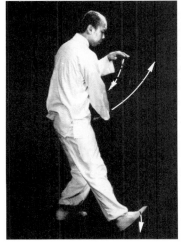

Illus. 21

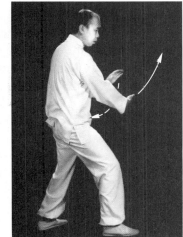

Illus. 22

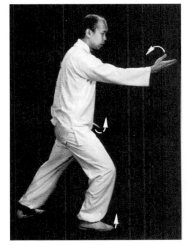

Illus. 23

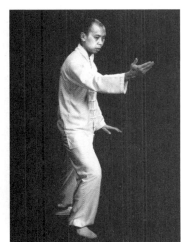

Illus. 24

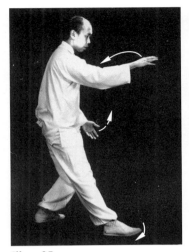

Illus. 25

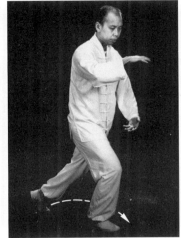

Illus. 26

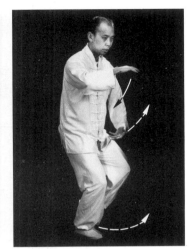

Illus. 27

Step 5 ▰▰▰▰▰▰▰▰▰▰▰ Using Illus. 25–27, repeat Step 3, from the opposite side.

Step 6 ▰▰▰▰▰▰▰▰▰▰▰ Using Illus. 28–30, repeat Step 4, from the opposite side.

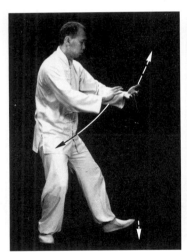

Illus. 28

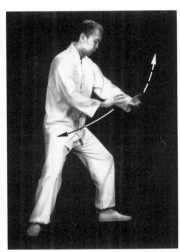

Illus. 29

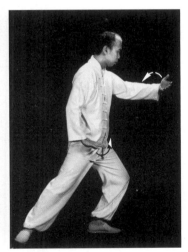

Illus. 30

Note ▰▰▰▰▰▰▰▰▰▰▰ Keep your upper body erect and your shoulders relaxed, your arms slightly bent (never straight). The turning of your upper body starts at your waist, the hips being the axis of rotation. The creation of "parting the mane" and the marksman position is done in a coordinated fashion and an even tempo; move your arms and legs in harmony. When stepping forward in the marksman position your heel should touch the floor first before your foot comes slowly to rest on its sole. With your toes pointing forward, do not bend your knee beyond the tips of the toes. Keep your leg relaxed, but do not straighten your knee. Your feet should be in a 40° to 60° angle to each other. If not, correct by turning the heel of your back leg.

In the marksman position your heels should not be in line. Your feet should rest on the left and right side of your body's midline, about 12 inches apart (Illus. 31).

Face east at the end of the sequence.

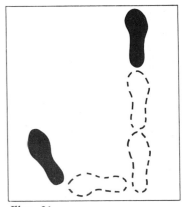

Illus. 31

Sequence 3: The Stork Spreading Its Wings (Bai-Ne Liang-Chi)

■■■■■ *Step 1*

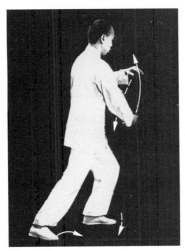

Illus. 32

Turn your upper body slightly to the left, with all of your weight on your left foot, while taking 1/2 step forward with your right foot.

Simultaneously, move your arms into the ball holding position, keeping your wrists and elbows relaxed (Illus. 32).

■■■■■ *Step 2*

Shift all your weight to your right foot while you turn your upper body to the right. Keep your hands in the ball holding position. Look at your right hand and bring your right foot forward, gently resting only the tips of the toes on the floor. This is the left "empty step" (Illus. 33).

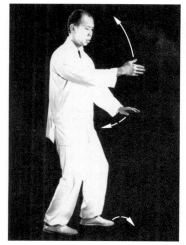

Illus. 33

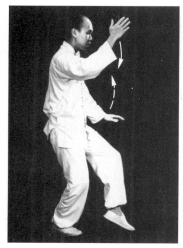

Illus. 34

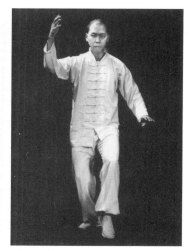

Illus. 35

As you take the empty step, turn your upper body slightly back to the left, moving your left hand down to your left hip and lifting your right hand up to your right temple (Illus. 34). Let your eyes follow this movement. Your left fingertips should point forward with the palm facing down. Your right fingertips should point up with the palm facing in. Look straight ahead at the end of the movement (Illus. 35).

Note It is essential to shift your weight and move your arms in harmony. Make sure at the end of the sequence your chest isn't pushed, your arms are relaxed, your left knee isn't locked, and your right leg is bent and supporting all your weight.

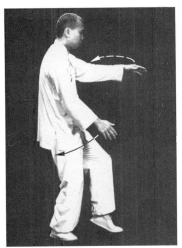

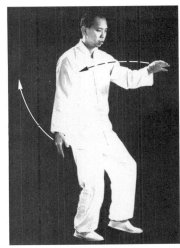

Sequence 4: Brush Your Knee and Step (Left and Right)
(Zuo-You Lu-Xi Niu-Bu)

Illus. 36   *Illus. 37*

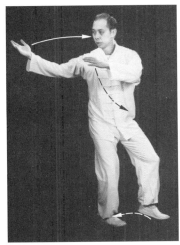

Illus. 38

Turn your upper body to the left. Move your right hand down in front of your body and your left in an arch upwards to the right side of your chest, palms facing down (Illus. 36).

Now move your upper body to the right, and bring your right arm, in an arch, up to ear level. Keep your palm facing upwards at an angle (Illus. 37).

Finally, bring the toes of your left foot, on the floor, next to your right foot. Bring your right hand to your ear and move your left hand down and outward (Illus. 38). Look first at your left, then your right hand.

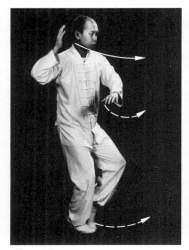

Illus. 39

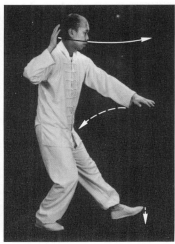

Illus. 40

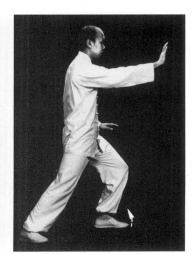

Illus. 41

Step 2 Turn your upper body left and take one step forward to the left, getting into the marksman position. Continue moving your left arm outward (Illus. 39).

Now bring your left arm up across your left knee to your left hip. Push your right hand, at ear level, forward, past your ear, until it's fully extended (Illus. 40).

Keep your left knee bent, your body weight mostly on the left foot, and your right knee relaxed. Your left palm should face down with fingertips forward. The right palm should face forward with fingertips upwards. Look at your right fingertips (Illus. 41).

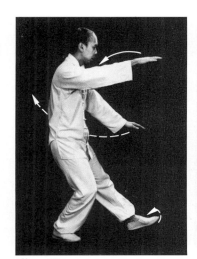

Illus. 42

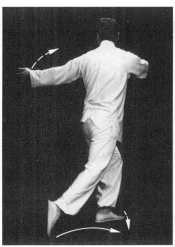

Illus. 43

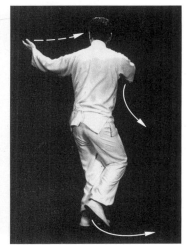

Illus. 44

Now, while slowly bending your right knee, shift your weight to your right foot. Lift your left foot slightly and turn your toes to the left. Turn your left palm upwards and move it in an arch, to ear level. Keep it close to your body. Your elbow will bend slightly and your palm will face upwards at an angle (Illus. 42). *Step 3*

Now turn your body farther to the left and begin to shift your weight from your right to your left foot. Touch the floor with your toe only and bring your right foot next to your left (Illus. 43).

Move your right hand, in an arch, to chest height, keeping your elbow bent slightly. Your palm should point down, and you should look at your left hand (Illus. 44).

Using Illus. 45 and 46, repeat Step 2 from the opposite side. *Step 4*

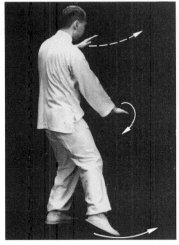 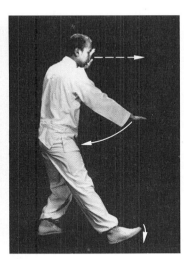 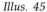

Illus. 45   *Illus. 46*

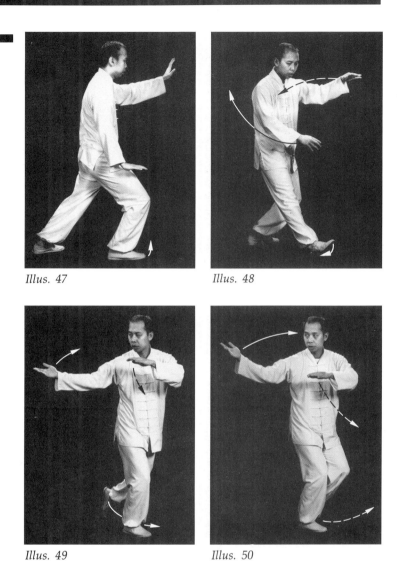

Illus. 47   *Illus. 48*

Illus. 49   *Illus. 50*

Using Illus. 47–50, repeat Step 3, from the opposite side.

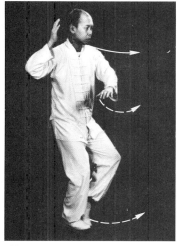

Illus. 51

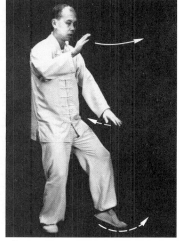

Illus. 52

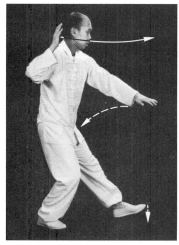

Illus. 53

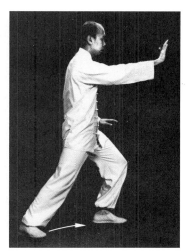

Illus. 54

Using Illus. 51–54, repeat Step 2.

Don't lean forward or backwards with your upper body while you move your hand forward. Relax your thighs, hips, and pelvis, and let your shoulders and elbows "hang loose." Relax your wrists and hands.

Note

Coordinate the movements of your hands, legs and thighs into a harmonizing whole. Remember, in the marksman position your toes should point forward, your feet 12 inches apart.

Face forward at the end of the sequence.

Sequence 5:
Playing the Lute
(Shou-Hui Pi-Pa)

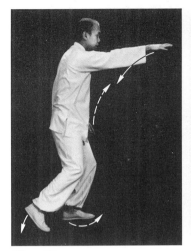

Illus. 55

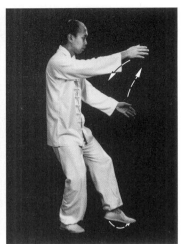

Illus. 56

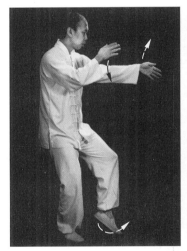

Illus. 57

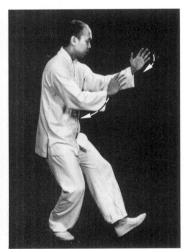

Illus. 58

Take one step forward with your right foot and let it support your weight. Turn your upper body about 20° to your right. Start to bring your right arm, in an arch, down and your left one, in an arch, up (Illus. 55). Lift your left heel off the floor, so that only the toes are touching, and continue moving your arms in (Illus. 56).

Now bend your right elbow and move your right hand first to your chest, then down towards your left elbow. Move your right hand up slightly (Illus. 57). Bring your left foot forward, into an empty step, and look towards your left index finger. Your elbows should be slightly bent, and your palms should face each other (Illus. 58).

Your weight is over your right foot at all times for good balance. Keep your upper body upright, and relax your chest. Do not pull your shoulders up and don't let your elbows stick out. Move your left hand in an arch upwards alongside your body and then forward. The same goes for your right hand. When moving your right foot forward a 1/2 step, touch the floor with the tips of your toes first, and then lower the rest of your foot. Shift your weight and move your hands in harmony.

Face east at the end of the sequence.

Note

Sequence 6:
Step Back and
Swirl Your Arms
(Left and Right)
(Zuio-You
Dao-Jun-Hong)

Step 1

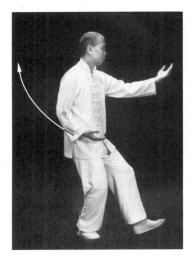

Illus. 59

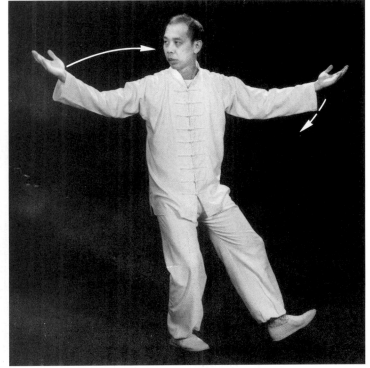

Illus. 60

Turn both your palms up and bring your right arm, in an arch, down across your chest to your hip. Bend your elbow slightly (Illus. 59).

Now slowly turn your body 45° to your right and bring your right arm, in an arch, upwards to shoulder level. Follow the turn of your body with your eyes, first to your right hand, then to your left. Simultaneously, bend your right elbow and bring your forearm up towards your face (Illus. 60).

Step 2

Take a step back with your left leg, your foot slightly off the floor. Continue moving your right forearm forward (Illus. 61). When your arm reaches ear level push your right hand straight forward, palm facing out. Move your left foot back with only your toes on the floor (Illus. 62).

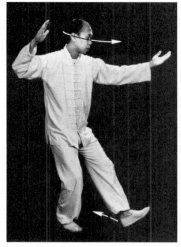

Illus. 61

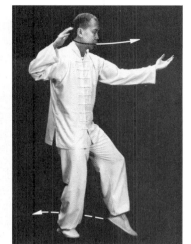

Illus. 62

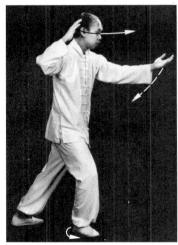

Illus. 63

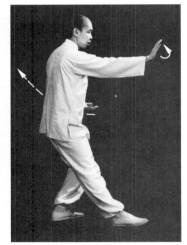

Illus. 64

Now start bringing your left hand, in an arch, downwards to your waist. Turn your right foot, on the toes, until it points forward (Illus. 63). Finish the right empty step, and move your left arm up to ear level. At the same, turn your right palm up. Look at your left, then straight ahead, focusing on your right hand (Illus. 64).

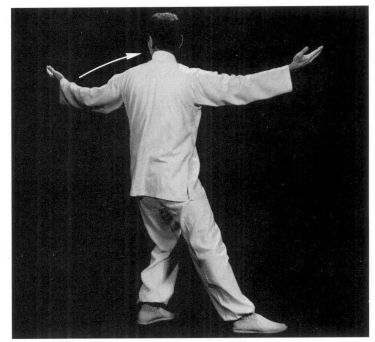

Illus. 65

Turn your upper body 45° to your left. Move your left hand, in an arch, in towards your ear. At the same time, turn your right palm upwards. Look first to your left, then straight ahead (again at your right hand) (Illus. 65).

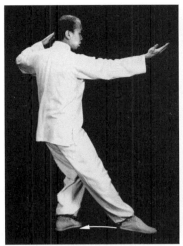

Illus. 66

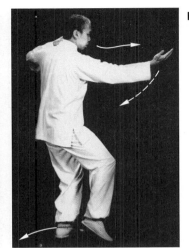

Illus. 67

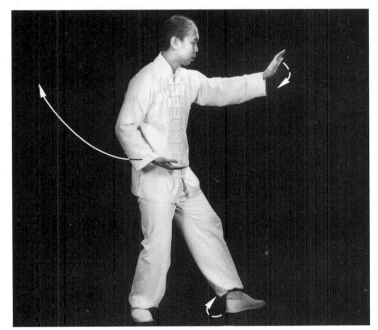

Illus. 68

Using Illus. 66–68, repeat Step 2, from the opposite side.

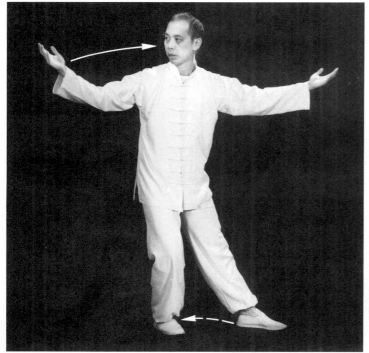

Illus. 69

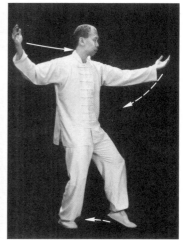

Illus. 70

Step 5 ■■■■■■■■■■■■ Using Illus. 69 and 70, repeat Step 3, from the opposite side.

Step 6 ■■■■■■■■■■■■ Using Illus. 71–73, repeat Step 2.

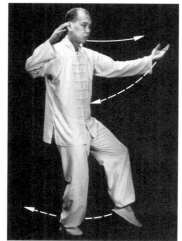

Illus. 71

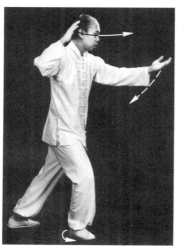

Illus. 72

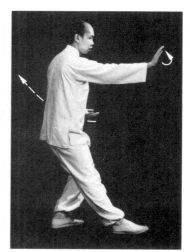

Illus. 73

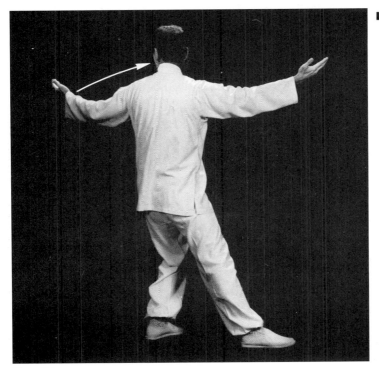

Illus. 74

Using Illus. 74, repeat Step 3.

Step 8 ━━━━━━━━

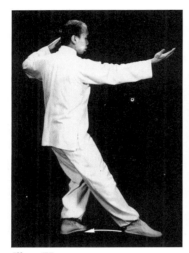

Illus. 75

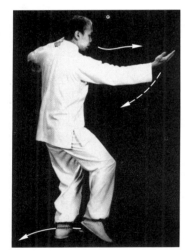

Illus. 76

Note ━━━━━━━━

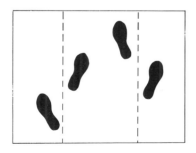

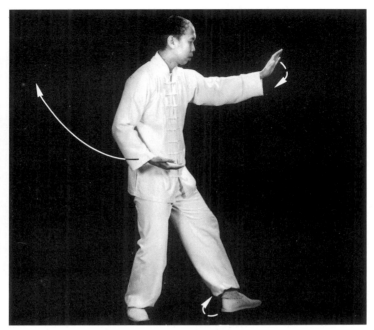

Illus. 77

Using Illus. 75–77, repeat Step 4.

Don't straighten your elbow when you push your arm forward or pull it back. Synchronize your body turns with your arm movements and keep your shoulders, waist, and hips relaxed. Your hand movements should be smooth and gentle.

To step backwards touch the floor with the tips of your toes and lower your foot slowly. At the same time, turn your front foot on the toes (as you turn your body) until it points forward. Your back foot should be positioned slightly outward from your front foot.

It is imperative that your feet are not in a straight line. The back foot should never cross your other foot (Illus. 78).

When you step back, look in the direction of your body's turn. Now, slowly, look forward and then back to the hand (on the other side of your body). Make your last step backwards with your right foot and make sure that the position of your toes is outward slightly.

Face east at the end of the sequence.

Illus. 78

Sequence 7: Grasping the Sparrow's Tail (Left) (Zuo Lan-Qiao-Wei)

Turn your upper body slightly to the right. At the same time move your right hand, in an arch, sideways and up to ear level. Keep your arm straight and your palm facing up. Your left palm should face forward and your eyes should be fixed on it (Illus. 79).

■■■■■■ *Step 1*

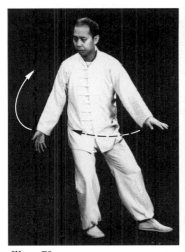

Illus. 79

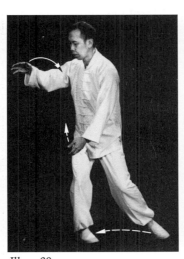

Illus. 80

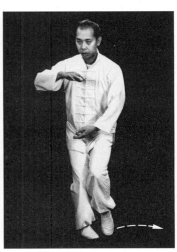

Illus. 81

Keep moving your upper body to the right. Now start to bring your left arm down and across your abdomen. Lower your right hand (Illus. 80).

■■■■■■ *Step 2*

Start to move your right hand in front of the right side of your chest, palm down. Simultaneously, shift your weight to your right foot. Turn your upper body slightly to the right as you pull your left foot to your right (Illus. 81). Bring your hands into the ball holding position, and pull your left foot next to your right, with only your left toes on the floor. Look at your right hand.

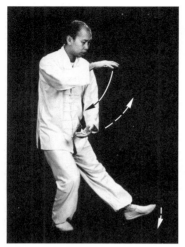

Illus. 82

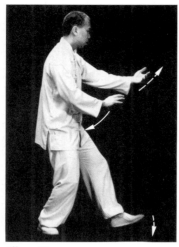

Illus. 83

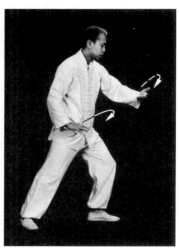

Illus. 84

Step 3

Start turning your upper body back to your left. Take one step forward and to your left with your left foot. Simultaneously, move your left hand forward to your left, elbow slightly bent and palm pointing in (towards you), and your right arm down towards your abdomen (Illus. 82).

Shift your weight to your left foot, bend your left knee, and stretch your right leg to get into the marksman position. At the same time, continue moving your hands until your left hand is at shoulder level, and your right hand goes, in an arch, past your hip and under your left wrist. This is called a *Peng* movement (Illus. 83). Make sure your weight is on your left leg and your eyes are on your left hand (Illus. 84).

Note

During the Peng movement relax your waist and keep your arms slightly bent. Coordinate moving into the markman position with turning your upper body. Your feet should be not more than 3 inches apart (Illus. 85).

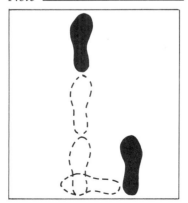

Illus. 85

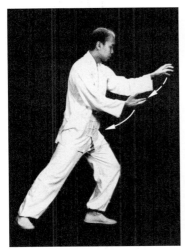
Illus. 86

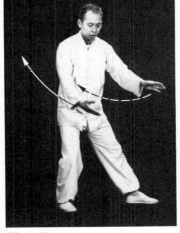
Illus. 87

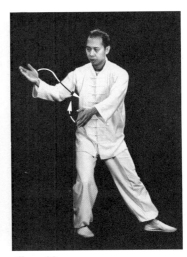
Illus. 88

Turn your upper body slightly to the left, facing east. Turn your left palm downwards and bring your arm forward a little. Start bringing your right arm down (Illus. 86).

Step 4

 Start to shift your weight over to your right foot and turn your upper body to the right. Simultaneously, move both arms, each in an arch, across your stomach (Illus. 87). Now bring your arms, still in an arch, up and backwards until your right hand is at shoulder level. Check to see that your left arm is slightly bent and in front of your chest. Your left hand should be in front of your right shoulder with your palm pointing back towards your body (Illus. 88). This is called a *Lu* movement.

During the Lu movement do not bend your upper body forward or push out your buttocks. When you turn your upper body you should move your hands as well. Keep your left foot flat on the floor when you shift your weight.

Note

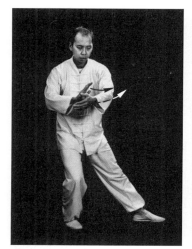

Illus. 89

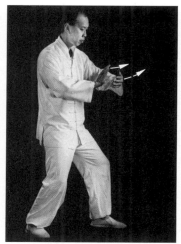

Illus. 90

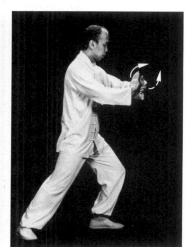

Illus. 91

Step 5   Start to turn your upper body back to your left, and bend your right arm, bringing your right hand inside your left wrist (Illus. 89). (There should be 2 inches between your left forearm and your right wrist.)

Now slowly move your hands forward and up to your shoulders, as if you wanted to push something away from you. Start to shift your weight to your left foot and go into the marksman position (Illus. 90). Bring your hands around so your left palm faces back, and your right one faces forward, left arm in the arch, right arm slightly bent. This is a *Ji* movement (Illus. 91). Look at your left wrist.

Note   During a Ji movement, make sure that your upper body remains erect. You should be pushing forward with your hands, turning your body and getting in the marksman position simultaneously. Look east (right) at the end of the Ji movement.

Step 6   Turn your palms down and cross your right hand over your left (Illus. 92).

Now move your right hand to the right, bringing it next to your left hand, palms still down. Start shifting your weight to the right and bring your hands a shoulder's width apart (Illus. 93). Lean backwards and lift your left foot, with only the heel touching the floor.

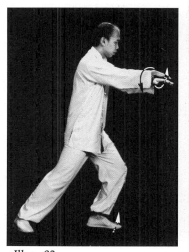
Illus. 92

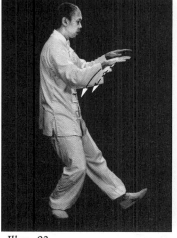
Illus. 93

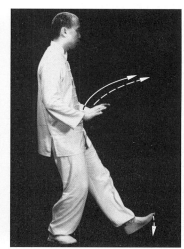
Illus. 94

With your palms still pointing down, bring both hands, in an arch, down to your abdomen; then, still in an arch, move them straight ahead (Illus. 94). Look straight ahead.

Step 7

Shift your weight back to your left foot, bend your knee and go into the marksman position. Your arms should be straight out in front of you, palms up, and you should be looking straight at them (Illus. 95). This is called an *An* movement.

Note

When you do the An movement push your hands up and forward in an arch. Bend your elbows slightly. Move your hands as you shift your weight and move into the marksman position.

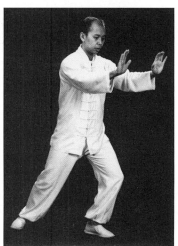
Illus. 95

Sequence 8: Grasping the Sparrow's Tail (Right)
(You Lan-Qiao-Wei)

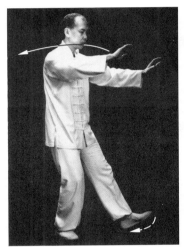

Illus. 96

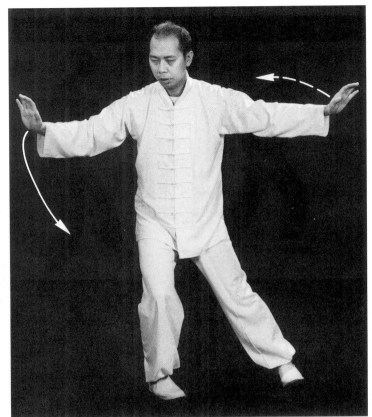

Illus. 97

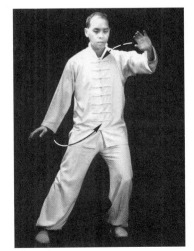

Illus. 98

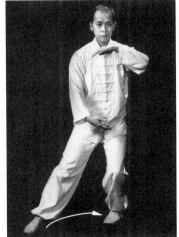

Illus. 99

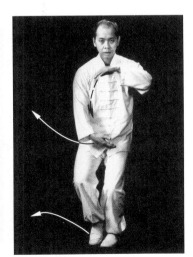

Illus. 100

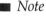

Shift your weight to your right foot and move your left foot inward (Illus. 96). Make an arch with your right hand to your right at shoulder level (Illus. 97). Now move your arm down and in front of your abdomen and turn your upper body to the right. Start to move your left arm up towards your face (Illus. 98).

Now shift your weight to your left and turn your left palm out, away from you. Begin bringing your hands into the ball holding position (Illus. 99). Rest your right foot on your toes, next to your left foot. Look to your right hand (Illus. 100).

Note

Turn the tips of your left toes as far as possible to your right. Your left foot should point to the southwest after the turn is completed.

Step 2

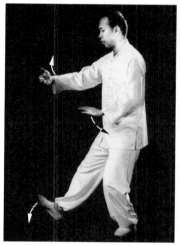

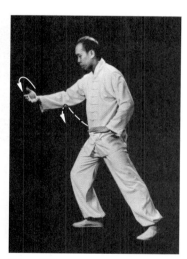

Illus. 101   *Illus. 102*

Using Illus. 101 and 102, repeat Step 3, Sequence 7, from the opposite side.

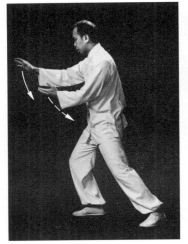

Illus. 103

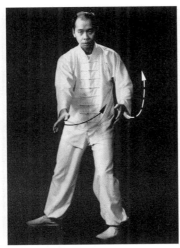

Illus. 104

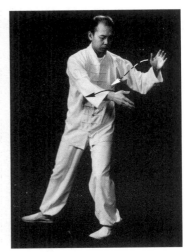

Illus. 105

Step 3  Using Illus. 103–105, repeat Step 4, Sequence 7, from the opposite side.

Step 4 Using Illus. 106–108, repeat Step 5, Sequence 7, from the opposite side.

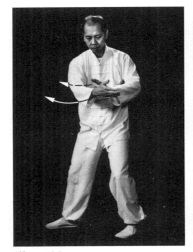

Illus. 106

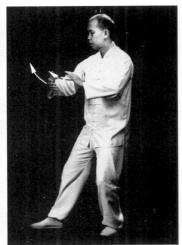

Illus. 107

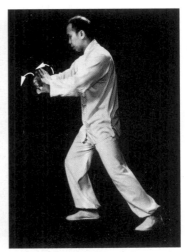

Illus. 108

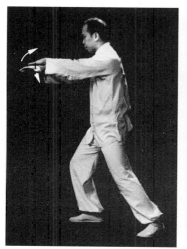

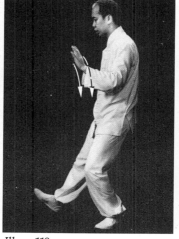

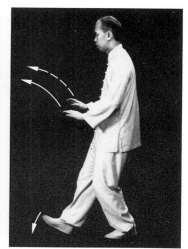

Illus. 109   Illus. 110   Illus. 111

Using Illus. 109–111, repeat Step 6, Sequence 7, from the opposite side.  *Step 5*

Using Illus. 112, repeat Step 7, Sequence 7, from the opposite side. 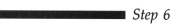 *Step 6*

Your position should be similar to the last position of Sequence 7. 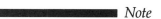 *Note*

Face west at the end of the sequence.

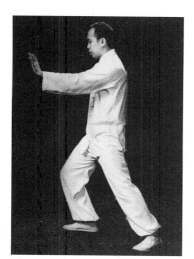

Illus. 112

Sequence 9:
The Whip
(Dan-Bian)

Step 1

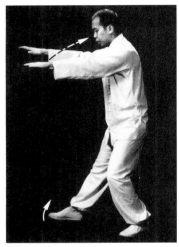

Illus. 113

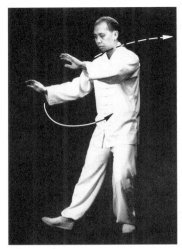

Illus. 114

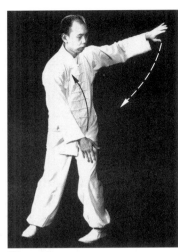

Illus. 115

Slowly shift your weight back to your left foot and move your left arm in an arch horizontally to your left (Illus. 113). Simultaneously, turn your upper body left, and bring your right toe, up and inward. Continue moving your left hand, and bring your right arm, in an arch, down across your abdomen (Illus. 114).

Continue turning your upper body to the left, and start to bring your left arm down to your left hip. Keep your elbow straight. Bring your right arm up to chest level (Illus. 115).

Note

Turn your right toes as far as possible to the left. Your right foot should point southeast after the turn.

Step 2

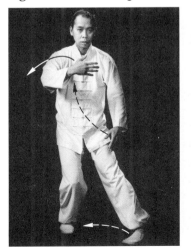

Illus. 116

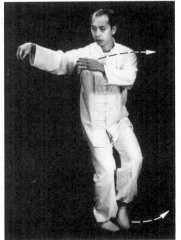

Illus. 117

Shift your weight back to your right foot and turn your upper body to the right, so you face south (Illus. 116). Position your left toes next to your right foot. Move your left arm, in an arch, up across your abdomen to chest level. Extend your right hand out, still at shoulder level, and form a hook with your right hand (Gou-Shou). Close your fingertips and relax your wrist. Look at your left hand (Illus. 117).

Turn your upper body to the left and take one step outward with your left foot (Illus. 118). Bring your left hand forward, at shoulder height, moving slowly and parallel to your body turn. Point your palm outward, away from you, and bring your right arm inward to ear level. Shift your weight to your left foot and go into the marksman position (Illus. 119).

 Step 3

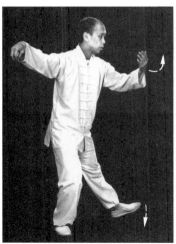

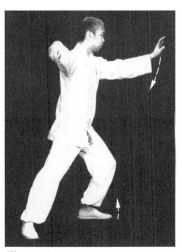

Illus. 118   Illus. 119

During this sequence keep your upper body erect and your waist relaxed. At the conclusion, bend both elbows down slightly and relax your shoulders.

Note

Move your left hand outward and push while you turn your body forward. Don't push and turn too fast or abruptly during the last phase of the body turn. Coordinate the transition from one movement to the next, and move in harmony.

At the end of the sequence your body and toes should point east northeast (about 15° from due east.) Your heels should be about 12 inches apart.

Sequence 10: Move Hands Like Clouds
(Yun-Shou)

Step 1 ▰▰▰▰▰▰▰▰

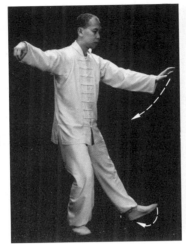

Illus. 120

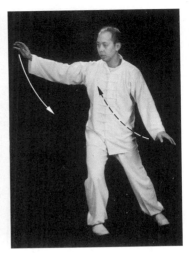

Illus. 121

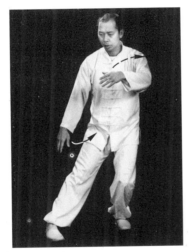

Illus. 122

First shift your weight to your right foot. Now move your left hand down and then up, in an arch, across your abdomen (Illus. 120). Start turning your upper body slowly to the right (southeast) and turn your left toes inward. Open your right hand and turn it so the palm faces outward and the tips of your fingers point up (Illus. 121).

Simultaneously, bring your left arm up across your abdomen to chest level, and bring your right arm down to your abdomen and up slightly. Look at your left hand (Illus. 122).

Do not move your right arm during this phase. It should only move because of your body's turning.

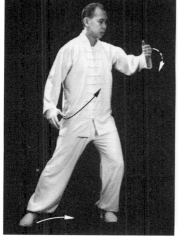

Illus. 123

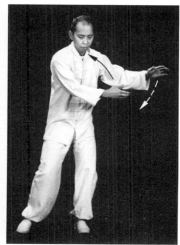

Illus. 124

Turn your upper body to the left (south southeast). Shift your weight slowly to your left foot. At the same time, continue the arch with your left hand from your face upwards to the left, then sideways, down to shoulder level (Illus. 123).

Now place your right foot parallel to your left foot, about 12 inches apart. Start your arm in an arch down and sideways to shoulder level. Slowly turn your palm outward. Simultaneously, move your right arm, in an arch, across your abdomen, and up to your left shoulder. Your palm should face your shoulder and be turned slightly sideways and up. Look at your right hand (Illus. 124).

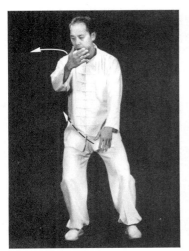

Illus. 125

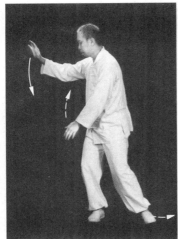

Illus. 126

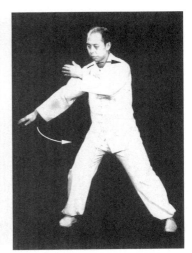

Illus. 127

Step 3 ████████████

Turn your upper body back to your right (south southwest) and shift your weight slowly to your right foot. Now make an arch with your right hand upwards to your right in front of the face and bring your left hand up across your abdomen (Illus. 125).

Now move your right arm, still in an arch, sideways to your right. Bring your left arm up to chest level, and take a wide step with your left foot sideways, about one and a half shoulder widths (Illus. 126).

Move your right arm down towards your abdomen, and your left arm out sideways. Look to your left hand (Illus. 127).

Step 4

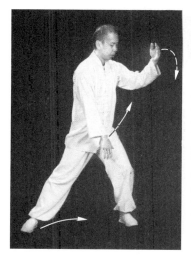

Illus. 128

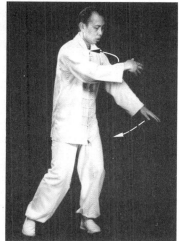

Illus. 129

Using Illus. 128 and 129, repeat Step 2.

Using Illus. 130–132, repeat Step 3.

Step 5

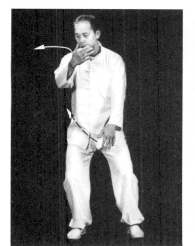

Illus. 130

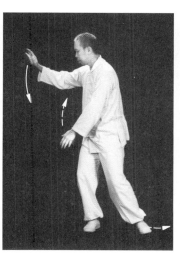

Illus. 131

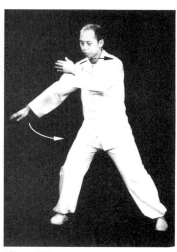

Illus. 132

Step 6 ▰▰▰▰▰▰▰▰▰▰▰▰▰▰▰▰▰   Using Illus. 133 and 134, repeat Step 2.

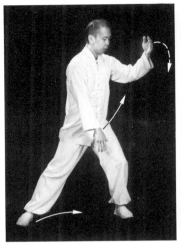 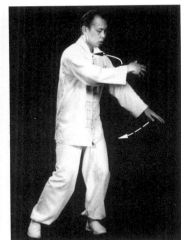

Illus. 133   *Illus. 134*

Note ▰▰▰▰▰▰▰▰▰▰▰▰▰▰▰▰▰   Your spine acts as an axis when your body is turning. Keep your waist and hips relaxed and don't pull your shoulder up. During the whole sequence make sure that the full leg remains bent. Keep your body steady, and don't bounce up and down.

Synchronize your arm's arch with the turn in your waist. The movement should be natural, round, and relaxed, in a slow and even tempo.

Keep your balance as you step sideways. Pay attention to the shifting of your weight from one foot to the other. Do not put the full weight on a foot until that foot is resting securely on the floor. Move your legs slowly and smoothly. Your toes should always point forward.

When your left or right hand crosses your face, watch the hand in motion. When you position your right foot next to your left, make sure that your right toes are turned inward slightly. This will prepare you for the next sequence.

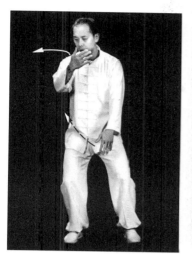

Illus. 135

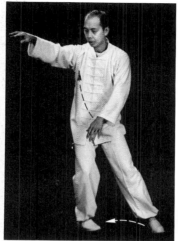

Illus. 136

Sequence 11: The Whip
(Dan-Bian)

Step 1

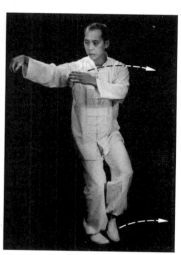

Illus. 137

Turn your upper body to the right. Shift your weight slowly to your right foot. At the same time, make an arch with your right hand from your face downwards and to the right (Illus. 135).

Lift your left heel so that only the toes touch the floor. Make an arch with your left hand, first downwards to your abdomen, then upwards and right to shoulder level. Extend your right arm out from shoulder level (Illus. 136).

Make a hook with your right hand, and start to move your left hand and foot, parallel to each other, outward. Look at your left hand (Illus. 137).

Step 2 Using Illus. 138 and 139, repeat Step 3, Sequence 9.

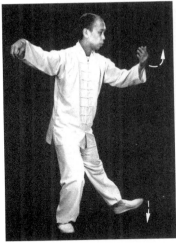

Illus. 138   Illus. 139

Sequence 12: Asking for Directions While Riding a Horse (Gao-Tan-Ma)

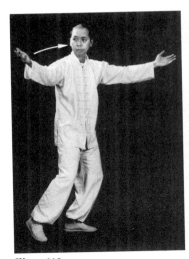
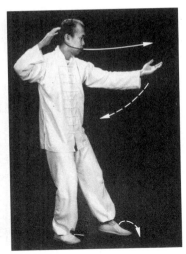

Illus. 140   Illus. 141

Step 1 Take a half step forward with your right foot as you open your right hand and turn both palms up. Slowly bend your elbows (Illus. 140). At the same time slowly turn your upper body to the right, and lift your left foot. Move your body back and slowly shift your weight to your right foot.

Raise your right hand to ear level and lift your left foot. Look first forward to your left and then to your right (Illus. 141).

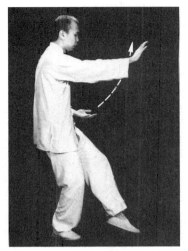

Illus. 142

Turn your upper body back to your left and look straight ahead. Move your left foot forward a little, letting only the toes touch the floor. (This is an empty step).

At the same time, move your left hand back to your left waist, palm up. Push your right hand forward. Your palm should now face forward, fingertips pointing up at eye level (Illus. 142). Look at your right hand.

Keep your upper body straight throughout the sequence. Relax your shoulders and bend your elbows slightly. Do not let your body bounce up or down when shifting your weight or changing steps.

Face east at the end of the sequence.

Note

Sequence 13: Right Heel Kick
(You-Deng-Jiao)

Step 1

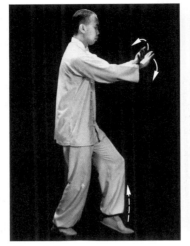

Illus. 143

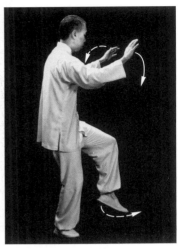

Illus. 144

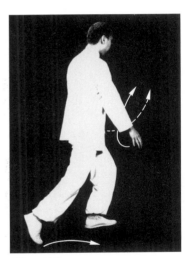

Illus. 145

Move your left hand forward so that it crosses your right, palms up. At the same time, step forward to your left with your left foot, touching the floor with your toes (Illus. 143).

Now move your hands apart sideways, in an arch. Turn your left palm down at an angle. Turn slightly outward and left (Illus. 144).

Shift your weight back to your left foot and bend your left knee. Extend your right leg and go into the marksman position. Look straight ahead (Illus. 145).

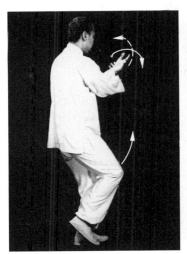

Illus. 146

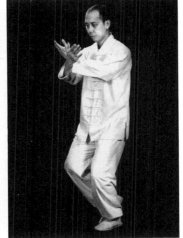

Illus. 147

Continue the arch with your hands and, at the same time, set your right toes next to your left foot (Illus. 146). Now bring your hands to your lower body and then up to chest level. Cross your hands, with both palms facing in, left over right. Look straight ahead (Illus. 147).

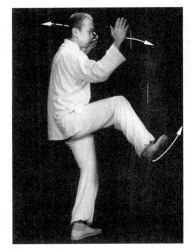

Illus. 148

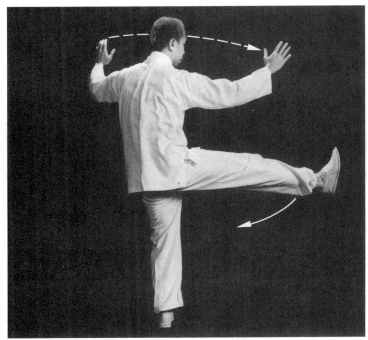

Illus. 149

Slowly turn your body to the right about 20°. Lift your right leg and bend your knee until your thigh is parallel to the floor. At the same time, spread both your hands, in an arch, from the cross outward (Illus. 148).

Slowly extend your foot forward to your right (outward) and continue to extend your arms out to shoulder level. Bend your elbows and face your palms forward. Look at your right hand (Illus. 149).

Note ▰▰▰▰▰▰▰▰▰▰▰

For good balance keep your upper body straight. When you cross your hands keep them about 12 inches in front of your chest. Keep your wrists at shoulder level during this movement. Bend your left knee a little when you extend your right foot for the heel push. Push forward from your heel.

Synchronize spreading your hands with pushing your right heel forward. At the end of the sequence your right foot should point southeast and your right arm should be parallel to your right leg.

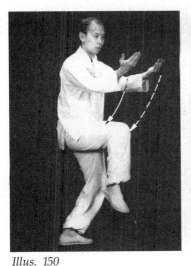

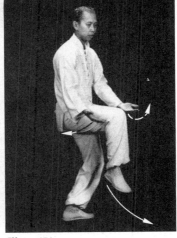

Sequence 14: Hit Your Opponent's Ears with Both Fists (Shuang-Feng Guan-Er)

Step 1

Illus. 150   *Illus. 151*

Bend your right knee 90°. Keep your thigh parallel to the floor and your toes pointing downwards. At the same time, bring your hands together; your left hand in an arch forward and up, then down, your right hand over to the left, until they are next to one another above your right knee (Illus. 150).

Turn both palms and guide both hands, in an arch, down to either side of your knee. Start to lower your knee slowly and move your hands away from each other (Illus. 151).

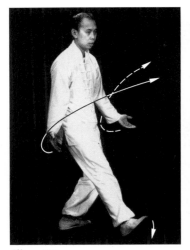

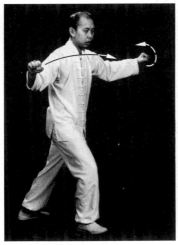

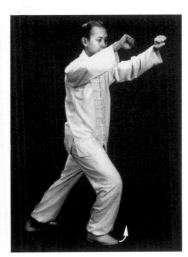

Illus. 152   *Illus. 153*   *Illus. 154*

Step 2 ■■■■■■■■■■■■■■■ Finish lowering your right foot until your heel touches the floor. Lower both hands and, in an arch, start to bring them back up (Illus. 152). Shift your weight to your right foot and go into the marksman position. Make fists with both hands and bring them towards each other when they reach chest level (Illus. 153).

Bring both fists in an arch up and forward to ear level, in front of your face. Point the knuckles of both fists upwards at an angle, about 8 inches apart. Look at your right fist (Illus. 154).

Note ■■■■■■■■■■■■■■■■■ At the conclusion of this sequence make sure that your head and upper body are straight, your hips, waist and shoulders are relaxed, and your elbows at a slight angle. Relax your fists and bend your arms in an arch. (Do not make "white-knuckle" fists.)

Your body and your fists should point in the same direction, southeast, the same as in the heel-push in Sequence 13.

The distance between your feet should not exceed 4 inches.

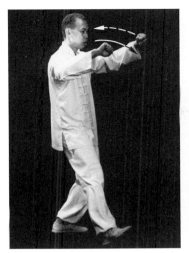
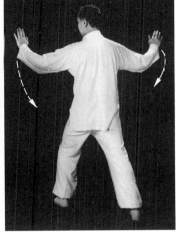

Sequence 15:
Left Heel Kick
(Zhuan-Shen
Zuo-Deng-Jiao)

Step 1

Illus. 155   Illus. 156

Step back, bend your left knee, and slowly shift your weight to your left foot. At the same time, open your fists and, in a gentle arch, move your hands apart and up (Illus. 155).

Now slowly turn your upper body to your left (north) and your right foot inward, the toes pointing east southeast. Bring your hands out sideways, and then start to move them down. Both your palms should face forward. Look at your left hand (Illus. 156).

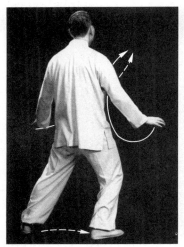

Illus. 157

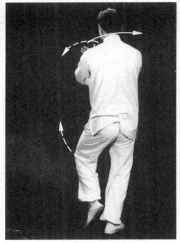

Illus. 158

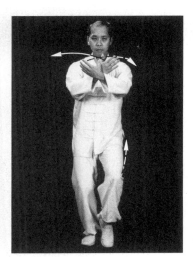

Illus. 159

Step 2 ▰▰▰▰▰▰▰▰▰ Slowly shift your weight back to your right foot and put your left foot on its toes, next to the right. Move your hands in an arch from the outside down, then inward and up (Illus. 157).

Cross your arms right over left, at chest level, with your palms facing your body. Look at your left hand and start to lift your left knee (Illus. 158, Illus. 159—front view).

Step 3 ▰▰▰▰▰▰▰▰▰ Gently turn your body to the left about 20°. Lift your left leg until the thigh is parallel to the floor. Start moving your hands outward at chest level (Illus. 160).

Slowly push your left foot forward to your left, until your whole leg is parallel to the floor (Illus. 161 and Illus. 162). Keep your elbows slightly bent downwards and your palms forward.

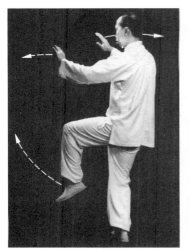

Illus. 160

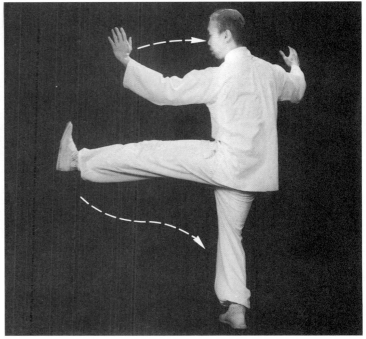

Illus. 161

This sequence follows the steps in Sequence 13, except from the opposite side.

At the end of this sequence your left foot should point northwest and create a 90° angle from your right leg.

Note

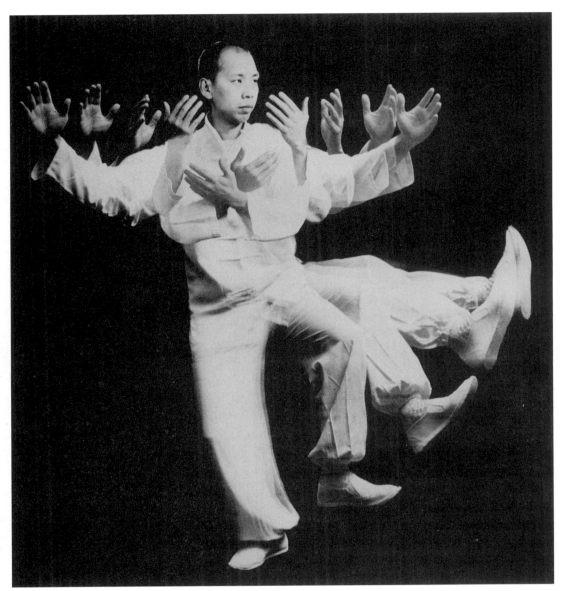

Illus. 162

Sequence 16: Climb Down and Stand on Your Left Leg
(Zuo-Xia-Shi du-Li)

Pull your left foot back. Keep your thigh in the horizontal position (your foot will float easily and loosely). Move your left hand, in an arch, up and then down slightly to shoulder level (Illus. 163).

Now make a hook with your right hand, and slightly turn your upper body to your right. Your left palm should face your shoulder, and you should look at your right hand (Illus. 164).

■■■■■ *Step 1*

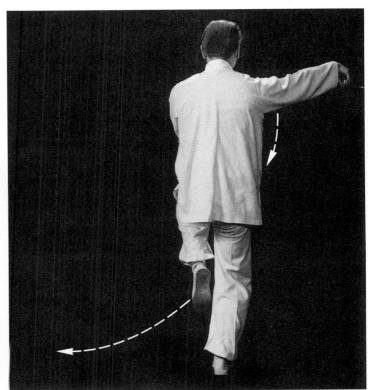

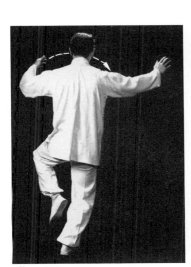

Illus. 163

Illus. 164

Step 2 ▰▰▰▰▰▰▰▰▰

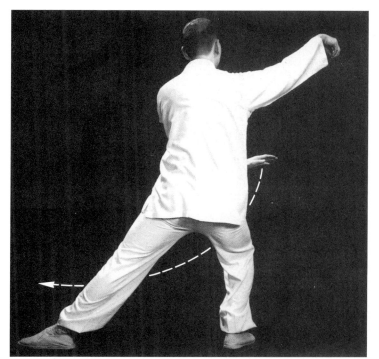

Illus. 165

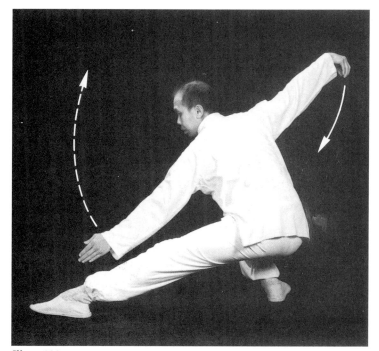

Illus. 166

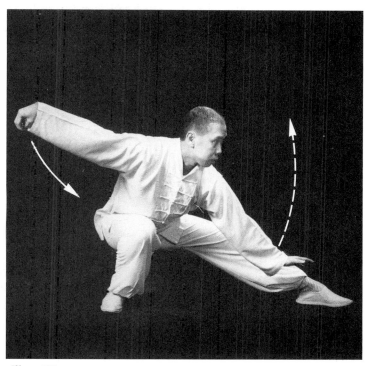

Illus. 167

Slowly bend your right knee and extend your left foot to your side, slightly touching the floor. At the same time, let your left hand "fall down" in an arch across the inside of your left leg (Illus. 165).

Now *slowly* lower your body as far as your right knee can bend. Do not force yourself too hard, your flexibility will improve over time. Finish the arch with your left hand by bringing it above your outstretched leg, and start to bring it up. Keep your right hand in the hook and start to bring it, in an arch, down to your hip (Illus. 166, Illus. 167—opposite view).

When you bend your right knee make sure that you don't lean too far forward. Stretch your left leg on the tips of your right toes; then let the soles of both feet rest flat on the floor. Form the axis of your body with the tip of your left foot and the heel of your right.

■ *Note*

Step 3 ▰▰▰▰▰▰▰▰▰▰▰ Turn your left toes outward as far as possible. Use your heel as the axis. Shift your weight to your left foot and bend your left knee. Extend your right leg and turn your toes inward. Slightly turn your upper body to the left. Raise yourself up with a forward movement as you shift your weight.

At the same time, move your hand left in an arch forward and up to shoulder level. Your palm should face inside. The right hand, formed into a hook, should face backwards. Slowly bring it down but keep it behind your body for the time being. Look at your left hand (Illus. 168).

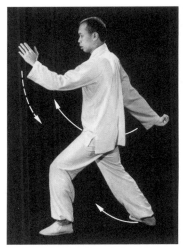

Illus. 168

Note ▰▰▰▰▰▰▰▰▰▰▰▰▰▰ Make sure that your left foot points straight ahead (west).

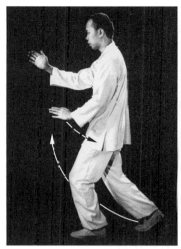
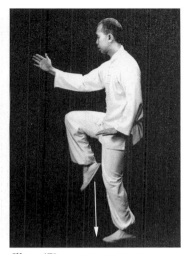

Illus. 169   *Illus. 170*

Start to bring your right foot forward, bending your knee. Finish the arch of your left hand by lowering it to your hip (Illus. 169).

At the same time, open your right hand from the hook and bring it, in an arch, up to shoulder level. The tip of the right elbow should be above the right knee, the fingertips pointing up and the palm inward.

Now raise your right foot off the floor, bending the knee fully. Look at your right hand (Illus. 170).

Bend your left leg slightly. Hang your right leg straight down and relax the ankle. Keep your upper body straight.

Note

Face west at the end of the sequence.

Sequence 17: Climb Down and Stand on Your Right Leg
(You-Xia-Shi Du-Li)

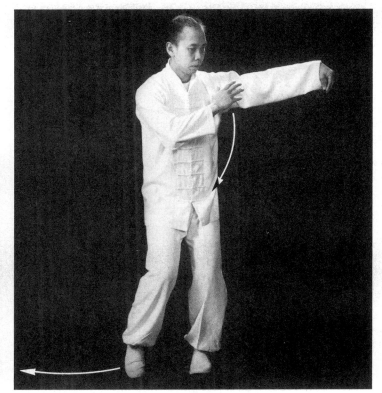

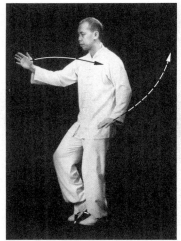

Illus. 171

Illus. 172

Step 1 ▰▰▰▰▰▰▰▰▰▰ Put your right toes in front of your left foot. At the same time, lift your left hand up to shoulder level. Make an arch with your right hand horizontally to your left shoulder (Illus. 171).

Spin your body slowly on your toes until you face south. Keep your weight on your left foot. Make a hook with your left hand and face your right palm up towards your shoulder at an angle. Look at your left hand (Illus. 172).

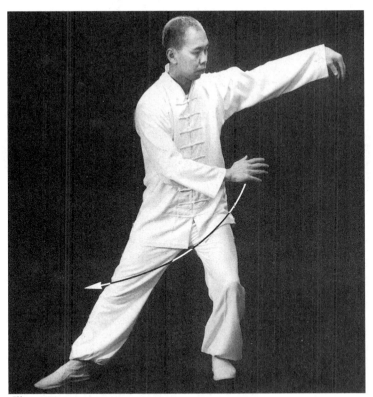

Illus. 173

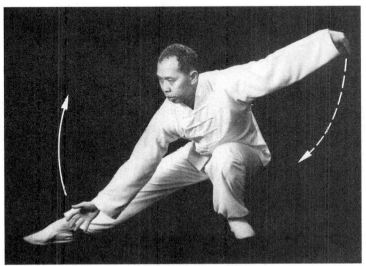

Illus. 174

Using Illus. 173 and 174, repeat Step 2, Sequence 16, from the opposite side.

Step 3

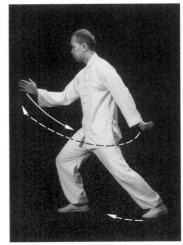

Illus. 175

Using Illus. 175, repeat Step 3, Sequence 16, from the opposite side.

Step 4

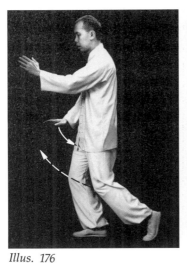

Illus. 176

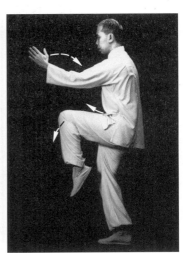

Illus. 177

Using Illus. 176 and 177, repeat Step 4, Sequence 16, from the opposite side.

Note

Make sure that your right toes touch the floor when you turn. Then gently lift your right foot, bend your knee, and stretch your right leg sideways on the floor.

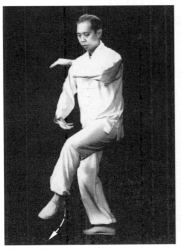

Illus. 178

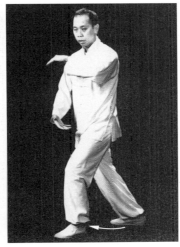

Illus. 179

Sequence 18: Throwing the Loom, (Left and Right) (Zuo-You Chaun-Zuo)

Step 1

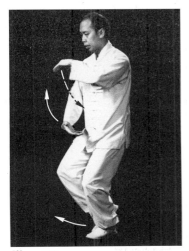

Illus. 180

Turn your body slightly to the left. Lift your left heel and put your left toe (pointed outward at an angle) in front of your right foot (Illus. 178). Bend both knees as if you wanted to sit down with your legs crossed. Move your hands into the ball holding position in front of your chest, left hand on top (Illus. 179).

Rest your right toes next to your left foot, and start bringing your left hand down and your right hand up (Illus. 180).

Keep your left foot next to your right.

Note

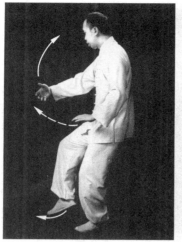

Illus. 181

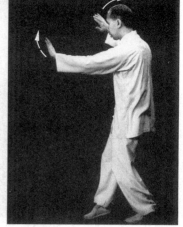

Illus. 182

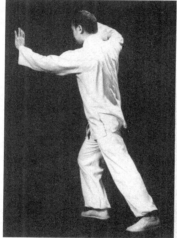

Illus. 183

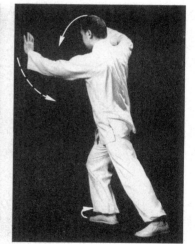

Illus. 184

Turn your body right and take one step forward with your right foot. At the same time, move your right hand, in an arch, up in front of your chest (Illus. 181). Bend your left knee and shift your weight to your right foot. Continue the arch of your right hand, bringing it up to your face and over to your right temple. Move your left hand up until it points outward and straight. Both palms should face forward (Illus. 182).

Move your feet into the marksman position, with your left hand extended at shoulder level and your right at your temple (Illus. 183). Your palms should face forward and your fingertips should point up. Look at your left hand (Illus. 184).

First, move backwards and shift your weight to your left foot. Then quickly shift it back to your right foot, and turn slightly to the right. At the same time, begin to move your hands into the ball holding position (Illus. 185).

Move your right foot next to the left, with only your right toes touching the floor. Finish moving into the ball holding position and look at your right forearm (Illus. 186).

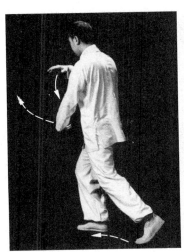 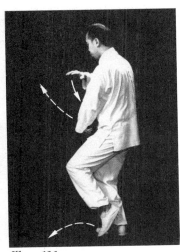

Illus. 185   *Illus. 186*

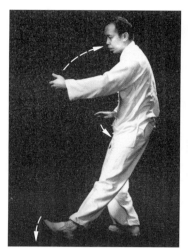

Illus. 187

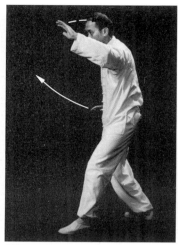

Illus. 188

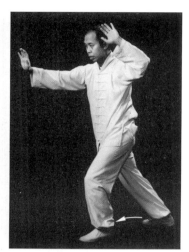

Illus. 189

Step 4 ▰▰▰▰▰▰▰▰▰ Using Illus. 187–189, repeat Step 2, from the opposite side.

Note ▰▰▰▰▰▰▰▰▰ Do not lean forward with your body during and after the hand movements. Relax your shoulders when you lift your hand. Synchronize your hand, leg, and body movements. The distance between your heels during the marksman position should be about 12 inches.

Face west at the end of Steps 2 and 4.

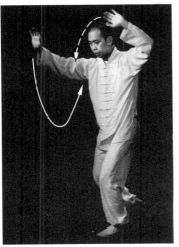

Illus. 190

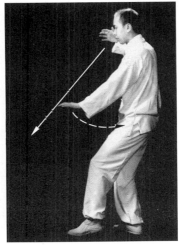

Illus. 191

Sequence 19: A Needle at the Bottom of the Ocean
(Hai-Di-Zhen)

Move your right hand, in an arch, down to your side, then slightly backwards and up, above your shoulder to ear level. As you move your right hand bring your left hand, in an arch, first forward then back, next to your left hip (Illus. 190).

At the same time, shift your weight to your right foot and take half a step with that foot. Position your left foot on the tips of the toes, and follow with a left empty step. Now turn your body slightly to the right (Illus. 191).

Now turn your body left and reach with your right hand forward and down. Your palm should face left and your fingertips should point down. Look at your right hand (Illus. 192).

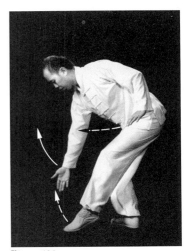

Illus. 192

Make your body movements small. Your upper body must be erect. Don't bend your head forward or push your buttock out. Bend your right leg deep, and your left leg moderately.

Face west at the end of the sequence.

Note

Sequence 20: Unfolding Your Arm Like a Fan
(Shan-Tong-Bi)

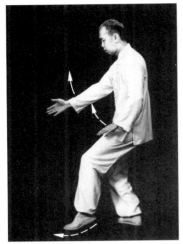 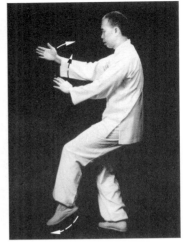

Illus. 193   *Illus. 194*

Lift your right arm upward and bend your elbow slightly. Begin to move your left hand, in an arch, upwards (Illus. 193). Continue moving both hands and, at the same time, bend your left knee and shift your weight to your right foot (Illus. 194). Turn your body slightly and take one step forward with your left foot.

Move your left hand in front of your body up to nose level, and your right hand to your right temple. Complete the step with your left foot (Illus. 195). Now move your left hand forward and out, and go into a left marksman position (Illus. 196). Your palms should face forward and your fingertips should point inwards. (Illus. 197). Look at your left hand (Illus. 198).

Note ■■■■■■■■■■■■ Relax your upper body, as well as your hips and waist. Do not fully extend your left arm and don't pull your shoulder muscles during the arch movements. Stretch your back muscles to move the arm. Synchronize your hand movements, your forward step, and your weight shift. The distance between your heels in the marksman position should not be more than 4 inches.

Face west at the end of the sequence.

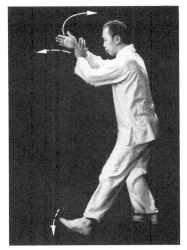

Illus. 195

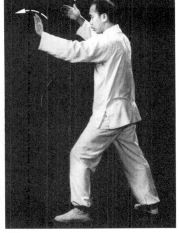

Illus. 196

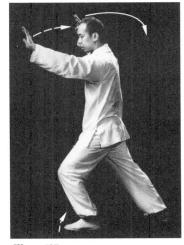

Illus. 197

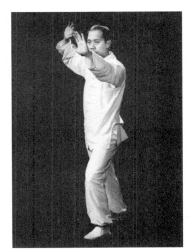

Illus. 198

Sequence 21: Turn Around, Ward Off, and Punch
(Zhuan-Shen Ban-Lan-Chui)

Step 1

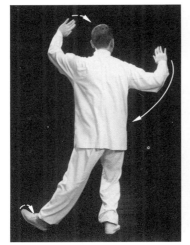

Illus. 199

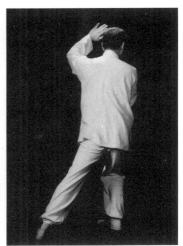

Illus. 200

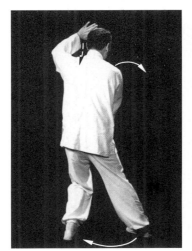

Illus. 201

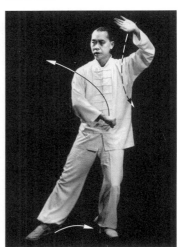

Illus. 202

Step back, shift your weight to your right foot, and turn your body 180° to your right. At the same time, make a wide arch with your right hand upwards, then downwards (Illus. 199). Move your left hand to your forehead, and move your right hand down to your lower chest (Illus. 200). As you do this, make a fist with your right hand, and move it past the left rib cage with the fist pointing down. Your left palm should face forward, and you should look straight ahead (Illus. 201—back view, Illus. 202—front view).

Note

Point your left toe north northeast.

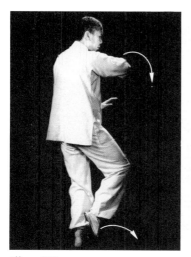

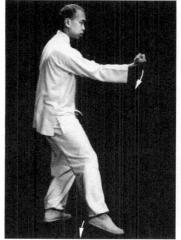

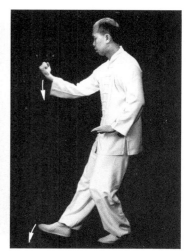

Illus. 203   *Illus. 204*   *Illus. 205*

Keep turning your body to the right (east). Lower your
left hand to your left hip, palm facing down and fingertips pointing forward. At the same time, move your fist
in front of your body (Illus. 203). The knuckles should
face down.

   Simultaneously, pull your right foot back next to your
left, and immediately take one step forward with your
right foot, letting only the heel touch the floor. Now
snap your fist forward and out, extending the arm full
(Illus. 204—right view, Illus. 205—left view). Look at
your right fist.

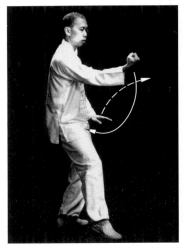

Illus. 206

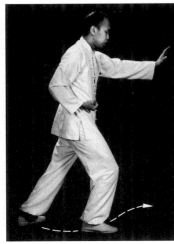

Illus. 207

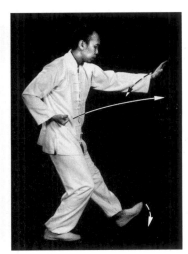

Illus. 208

Step 3 Move your right fist, in an arch, back to your right waist. Begin to bring your left hand up (Illus. 206).

At the same time, slowly shift your weight to your right foot and take one step forward with your left (only your heel should touch the floor). Push your arm forward, with your palm facing downwards and your fingertips pointing upwards (Illus. 207).

Start to lower your left foot and look to your left hand (Illus. 208).

Note When "warding off" with your left hand, keep the elbow slightly bent.

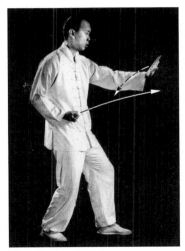
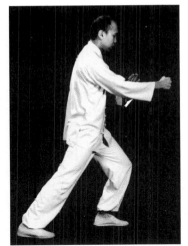

Illus. 209   *Illus. 210*

Simultaneously, shift your weight to your left foot, bending the knee, and punch your right fist forward at chest height. The bottom of your fist should face inward (Illus. 209).

Pull your left hand back next to your right forearm, near the elbow. Look at your right fist (Illus. 210).

Note

Keep your fingers relaxed, and don't make "white knuckle" fists. When you move your right fist go slightly inward first, then do a slow arch outward. Stop next to the right side of your waist. Turn your fist inward and then outward. When you punch forward with your right fist, let your shoulder move slightly forward, but keep both your shoulder and elbow loose and hanging down.

The distance between your heels in the marksman position should be 4 inches.

Face east at the end of your upper body movement.

Sequence 22: Closure
(Ru-Feng Si-Bi)

Step 1

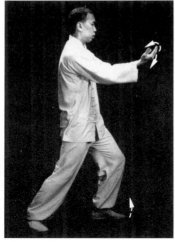

Illus. 212

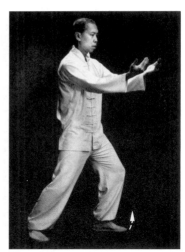

Illus. 213

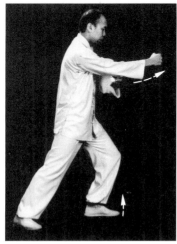

Illus. 211

Bring your left hand under your right elbow, palm up, and move it forward gently under your lower arm, as you open your fist (Illus. 211). At the same time, move your body back, shift your weight to your right foot and raise your left toes (Illus. 212).

Simultaneously, turn your right palm up. Move your hands away from each other and pull them slowly back towards your chest. Look straight ahead (Illus. 213).

Step 2

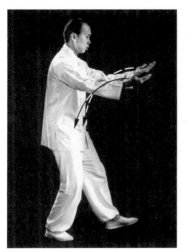

Illus. 214

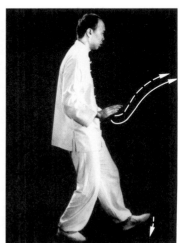

Illus. 215

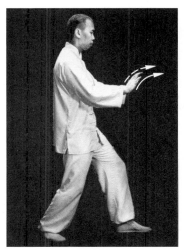

Illus. 216

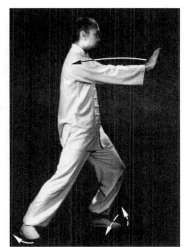

Illus. 217

As you turn both palms down, lower both your hands to your abdomen (Illus. 214). Now move them up again until both your wrists are chest high. Your palms should face forward, fingertips up (Illus. 215).

At the same time, shift your weight back to your left foot, lower your toes to the floor, and bend your left knee. You should be in the marksman position (Illus. 216). Start to bring your hands back (Illus. 217).

Keep your upper body straight and as you move back be sure that your buttock does not stick out. Synchronize shifting your weight to your right foot with moving your hands to your chest.

Bend your elbows slightly and keep them away from your body. Your hands should be a shoulder's width apart.

Face east at the end of the sequence.

■ *Note*

Sequence 23:
Cross Your Hands
(Shi-Zi-Shou)

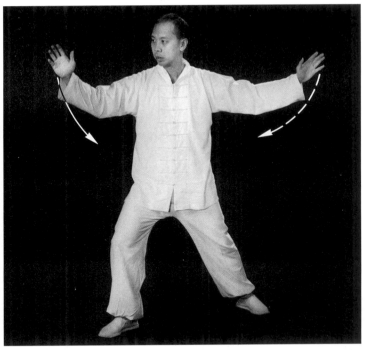

Illus. 219

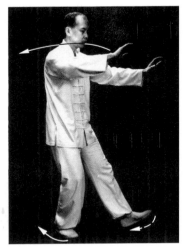

Illus. 218

Step 1 ▆▆▆▆▆▆▆▆▆▆▆ Move back and shift your weight slowly to your right foot, bending your knee. Continue bringing your hands back (Illus. 218). As you do this, slowly turn your body to the right. The toes of your right foot should point outward slightly, your left foot inward. Your hands should be at shoulder level, elbows bent slightly downwards, palms forward and fingertips pointing to the side (Illus. 219).

Note ▆▆▆▆▆▆▆▆▆▆▆ Turn your left toes inward as far as possible, so that they point south.

Step 2 ▆▆▆▆▆▆▆▆▆▆▆ Bring both arms, in an arch, down and across your abdomen, then upwards until they cross each other at chest height (Illus. 220). At the same time, slowly move your weight back to your left foot, turn your right toes inward and pull your right foot back to the left. Both feet will be next to each other, a shoulder's width apart. Lower your thighs until your knees are slightly bent (Illus. 221).

As you cross your hands, your wrists should be at

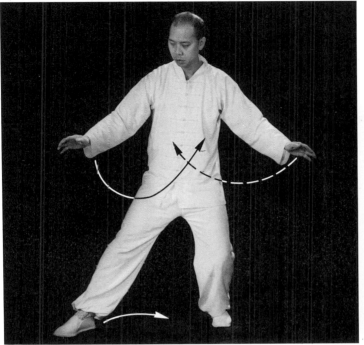

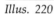

Illus. 220

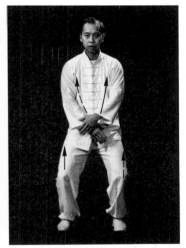

Illus. 221

shoulder level, your left hand should be between your body and your right hand. Both your palms should face you (Illus. 222). Look straight ahead.

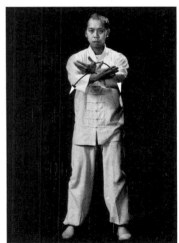

Illus. 222

Keep about 10 inches between your chest and your crossed hands. Bend your elbows slightly, so that your arms are nicely rounded. Let your shoulders hang down and hold both forearms away from your body. Do not lean forward with your upper body. When you straighten your knees, your body should be erect and your head should not lean forward or back.

Face south at the end of the sequence.

Sequence 24: Conclusion
(Shou-Shi)

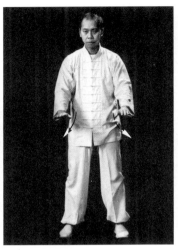

Illus. 224

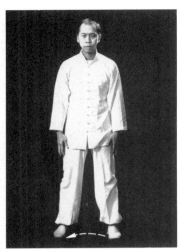

Illus. 225

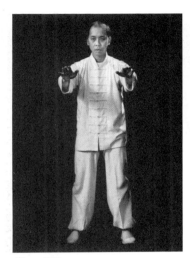

Illus. 223

Move both your hands outward (Illus. 223). With your palms facing down and your fingertips pointing forward, let them slowly fall down next to your hips (Illus. 224).

Move your feet together and look straight ahead (Illus. 225).

Note ▰▰▰▰▰▰▰▰▰▰▰

When you move your hands to your hips, relax your whole body and exhale a little longer than usual, so the Qi can "fall down deeply into the Dan-Tian (see p. 17).

Your hands should hang naturally next to your hips, facing inward. Both elbows should be limber and natural.

Conclude your tai chi ch'uan with a little walk, maybe around the room where you're working. This will add to the feeling of well-being.

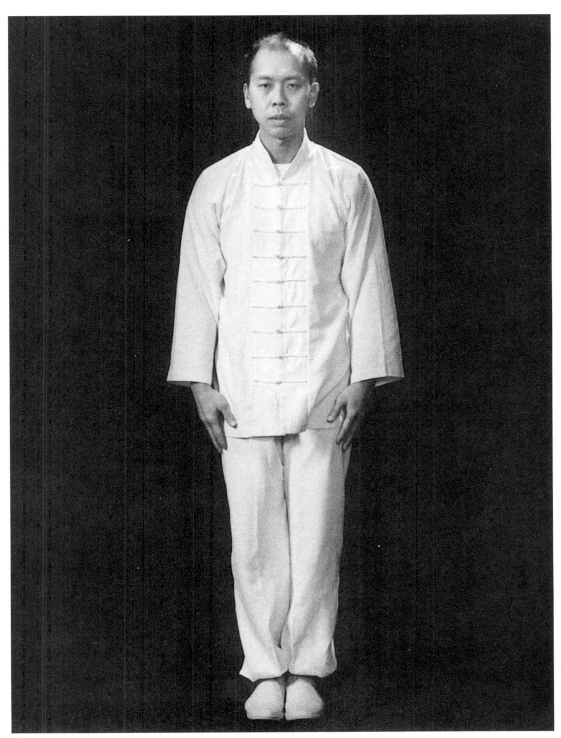

Illus. 226

Overview

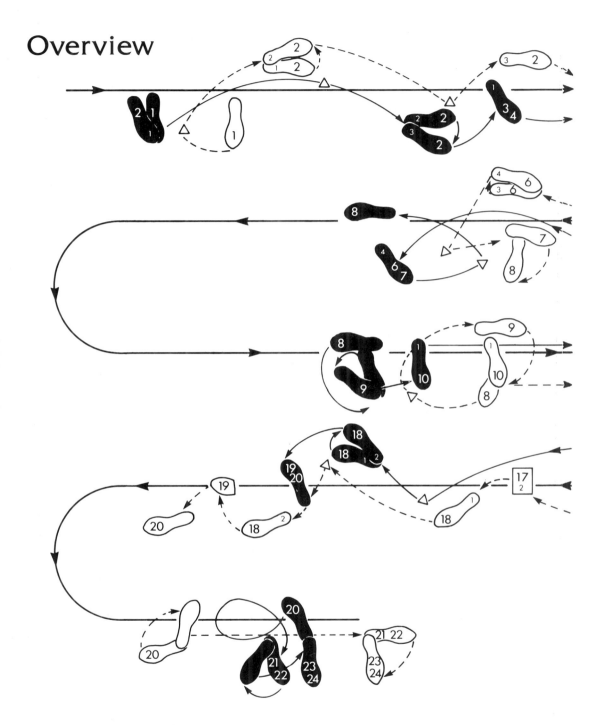

Diagram of the movement and position of the feet from the first to the twenty-fourth sequence.

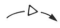 *Indicates at which point the ball of the foot is set on the floor during changes.*

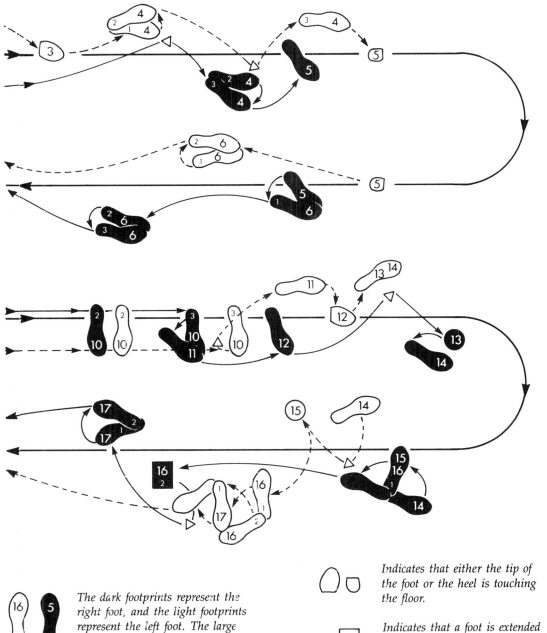

 The dark footprints represent the right foot, and the light footprints represent the left foot. The large numerals indicate the position of the feet during the respective sequences: the small numerals indicate the repetition of the sequences. Those diagrams without numerals indicate the change from one sequence to another.

Indicates that either the tip of the foot or the heel is touching the floor.

Indicates that a foot is extended in the air with the thigh parallel to the floor.

Indicates that during heel-push a foot is lifted off the floor by stretching the upper and lower leg.

The History and Effects of Tai Chi Ch'uan

Origin and Development

There are many different tales of tai chi ch'uan's begin-
nings and development. One version has it that Zhang
San-Feng had a dream on the Holy Mountain Wu-
Dang, during which the legendary Emperor Xuan-Wu
told him about tai chi ch'uan. Thus tai chi ch'uan was
a gift from the gods. Today we know that in the 17th
century tai chi ch'uan was developed by the Chen
family in the He-Nan Province of China. However, the
present form has come through many changes since
then. Chang-Quan ("long boxing") was handed down
by Chen Wang-Ting. It was named after the Chang-Jiang
River, the longest in China, because the movements
looked like the endlessly moving and flowing waters.

Chang-Quan consists of thirteen basic movements,
and is still called the "Thirteen Form" (Shi-San-Shi).
The eight basic hand movements and the five basic foot
movements are very much like the art of self-defense
develped by Qui Ji-Guang (1528–1587), a general of the
Ming Dynasty. He illustrated this art in the *Quan-Jing*,
(*Book of Boxing*). This was a synthesis of the then existing sixteen different schools of boxing (Family of Boxing). Thus, Qui Ji-Guang created a new form by con-
densing, selecting, and changing certain movements
and sequences. It has been suggested that tai chi ch'uan
had its origin in this style of fighting.

Wang Zong-Yuo (1736–1795), a master in the art of self-
defense, described this new boxing style in his book
Tai-Ji-Quan-Lun, a Discourse in Tai Chi Ch'uan. He empha-
sized, among other things, the connection between this
new school of boxing and the philosophy of Ying-Yang.
He gave it the name tai chi ch'uan.

From 1850 on, tai chi ch'uan quickly spread from the
He-Nan province throughout China, although many
profound changes took place along the way. The most
explosive and forceful elements were taken out. What
remained were the gentle and relaxing movements, and
they remain, to this day, the accepted form.

Tai chi ch'uan is used not only by athletes but also
by children, senior citizens and even the frail, because

111

it is so easy to do. It can also be used to prevent and treat illness and increase good health.

Forms and Styles

Tai chi ch'uan can take any of three forms.

The Large Form (Da-Jia)

This form uses natural and straight body posture and flowing, but brisk, movements that balance between agility and steadiness.

The Medium Form (Zhong-Jia)

This form can be distinguished by its distinct movements as well as a moderate posture. Its Chinese symbol is: 吴

The Small Form (Xiao-Jia)

Short range, quick, and agile movements are characteristic of this form. The Chinese symbol is: 武

There are five styles (or "schools") of tai chi ch'uan:

The Chen Style

The Chen style has the longest tradition. The smooth changes between movements, executed either with or without any force make this style unique. The change from sudden to slow and gentle movements is never abrupt but always smooth, as if it were done underwater. This style is also called Loa-Jia (The Old Form). This school incorporates all three forms.

The Yang Style

This style is the most popular inside and outside China. It was founded by Master Yang Lu-Chan, who was a student of Master Chen Chang-Xing of the Chen School. The new style, which he developed from the Chen, was further refined and arranged by his grandson Yang Cheng-Fu. It is a style characterized by quiet, smooth, harmonious and steady flowing movements, giving it an overall wavelike appeerence. This accounts for the popularity among the tai chi enthusiasts.

The Chinese symbol for this style is: 武

The Wu Style

Wu Yu-Xiang, this style's founder, was first a student of Master Yang Lu-Chan of the Yang style and later became a student of the Master Chen Qing-Ping of the Chen School.

A later Master of this school, Hao Wei-Zhen, was most responsible for the continued developement of this style. This is why this school is often called the Hao Style.

The movements are nimble and quick with only a small range and a flowing change between the opening and closing of the arms. All movements follow each other closely.

The Sun Style

The method of this style is similar to the Wu Style. Its founder was Master Sun Lu-Tang, who was a student of Master Hoa Wei-Zhen. He developed a whole new style, using many elements from various other boxing schools. Its trademarks are quick movements of the hands and feet as well as harmonious changes between backwards and forward movements. This is why it is sometimes called "the form of the flowing steps" (Huo-Bu-Jia).

The Chinese symbol is: 吴

The Manchu Wu Style

This school was founded by Master Quan-You from Manchu, and his son Jian-Quan, who later took the name of Wu. Quan-You was a student of Yang Lu-Chan who together with his son Yang Ban-Hou, formed the Yang Style. Quan-You also studied with Wu-Xiang, the founder of Wu-School. This style, like the Yang style, is known for its gentle and harmonious movements with flowing changes and a moderate posture, giving the impression of simplicity and tranquility.

These five styles represent the total tai chi ch'uan system which developed out of the different families. Every style carries its own specialties, but, since they are so closely related, they are much alike. It is, therefore, not difficult for a student of one style to become efficient in another, and, with little effort, one can change from the large to the medium to the small form. The choice of school depends entirely on constitution, preference, age and need. Beginners, however, should start with a simple system.

In 1956 the Sports Committee of the People's Republic of China developed tai chi ch'uan to accommodate people who were interested in this activity. The result was a shortened version of the Yang style, the so-called Peking Form, with 24 sequences. In 1957 a long form was added, with 88 sequences.

The shortened Peking Form is very popular, not only in China but in many foreign countries as well. The simplified posture and the logically developed degree of difficulty makes it an easy exercise, and it keeps the therapeutic value of its ancestors. The chart on page 115 gives an overview of the relationships, developments, and the important Masters of the tai chi ch'uan styles.

The Development of Tai Chi Ch'uan Styles

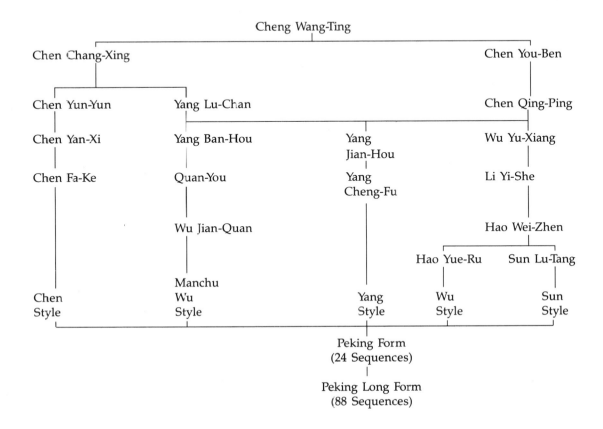

Cheng Wang-Ting

Chen Chang-Xing   Chen You-Ben

Chen Yun-Yun   Yang Lu-Chan   Chen Qing-Ping

Chen Yan-Xi   Yang Ban-Hou   Yang Jian-Hou   Wu Yu-Xiang

Chen Fa-Ke   Quan-You   Yang Cheng-Fu   Li Yi-She

Wu Jian-Quan   Hao Wei-Zhen

Hao Yue-Ru   Sun Lu-Tang

Manchu

Chen Style   Wu Style   Yang Style   Wu Style   Sun Style

Peking Form
(24 Sequences)

Peking Long Form
(88 Sequences)

The Effects of Tai Chi Ch'uan on the Human Body

The value of exercise in preventing and treating illnesses has been known in China for a long time, but only recently did the Research Institute for Sports Medicine in Peking examine the value of tai chi ch'uan. Eighty-eight people participated, ranging in age between 50 and 89. Thirty-two of them had long experience in the practice of tai chi ch'uan, the rest had none. The research showed that people with an active involvement in tai chi ch'uan were in far better shape. Their heart and circulatory function, their breathing and metabolic function, as well as the strength of their bone structure were far superior to those who did not pursue any physical activity other than their everyday normal routine.

The Nervous System

The central nervous system is responsible for the coordination of movements, balance and the workings of the heart, lungs, and other internal organs. When practising tai chi ch'uan, pay particular attention to "a quiet heart and a purpose of will." Be serene and composed when practising, and perform all movements with full mental alertness. This concentration will put aside distracting thoughts. When we do that, we use only a small area of the brain. This in turn gives the body a chance to recover from fatigue and stress by totally focusing on the sequences of the tai chi ch'uan movements. We also train our skills for better concentration.

Tai chi ch'uan requires a coordination of different parts of the body (like arms, legs, and eyes). Some sequences are complicated, but if you do them diligently you will allow the central nervous system to better support your body functions. Tai chi ch'uan will also have a very positive influence on your frame of mind, whether you do the whole form or only a few sequences. An improvement in the mental and physical state will be the reward, including your ability to react. There is a positive correlation between a healthy mind and a healthy body, and the renewed zest you will feel at the end of the session will also make you more fit.

People with chronic illnesses have been able to improve their condition with tai chi ch'uan. Through this therapy, they accepted responsibility for their own well-being. In every case, an improvement, if not a cure, was achieved.

Respiratory System

It is much more difficult to breathe when you are tense, because your chest, back, shoulders, or arms are tight. Tai chi ch'uan cures this by requiring attention to posture: relax your shoulders, keep your head and upper body straight, and "hang loose" without being limp. This will keep tension out of the chest area and help focus our concentration on the awareness of Dan-Tian (see p. 17).

Remember, Dan-Tian influences a breathing technique that intentionally involves the conscious use of the diaphragm.

Do not allow your breathing to become labored. It is more important in the beginning that breathing be quiet, deep, slow, even and gentle, and in harmony with the movements.

The specific posture and the deliberate breathing, as well as the calm and harmonious moving that tai chi ch'uan teaches, also increase the lungs' capacity and elasticity. If tai chi ch'uan is practised over a longer period of time, this will become obvious, and there will be less shortness of breath after physical exercises.

Blood Circulation

Tai chi ch'uan also influences the blood circulation in a very positive way.

The nervous system nourishes the heart and controls the way it pumps blood. Therefore, an improved nervous system will result in a better functioning heart.

Likewise, breathing that makes full use of the diaphragm positively affects the abdomen. The more the diaphragm is involved in the breathing process, the more effective the flow of blood will be through the circulatory system. The result is an overall improvement in well-being.

In addition, because the load on the muscles, joints, and walls of the arteries is so gentle during tai chi ch'uan, lower blood pressure and a better functioning

117

lymphatic system are also possible. The overall result is a much lighter workload for the heart.

People with many years of tai chi ch'uan experience show a much more efficient heart function, have lower blood pressure and suffer less often from arteriosclerosis when compared to people without tai chi ch'uan experience.

Digestion

Here again, the influence of tai chi ch'uan on the central nervous system shows a positive effect on the functions of the digestive system, especially its ability to absorb nutrients. Tai chi ch'uan breathing acts like a mechanical massage of the digestive system. These both aid blood circulation and add to the system's ability to function better. For this reason tai chi ch'uan is an excellent means of treatment and prevention of digestive diseases.

Metabolism

Today there is very little research on the advantages of tai chi ch'uan on the metabolic system. However, clinical observations make it safe to assume that the nervous system, functioning as a regulator, has a positive influence, similar to the one observed in the digestive system. Likewise, diaphragmatic breathing, which results in better blood circulation, positively affects the functioning of the liver and kidneys.

As with other body functions, the gentle and harmonious movements of tai chi ch'uan can improve the function of the metabolic system. Tai chi ch'uan, when practised for only a few months, can substantially decrease the concentration of globulin and cholesterol in the blood, and increase the concentration of protein.

The Muscular System

Tai chi ch'uan pays special attention to the posture. The spinal column is erect and the pelvis turned slightly forward and up (Illus. 5, p. 21). The lower vertebrae (located between the lowest rib and the pelvis) are vertically lined up with the back portion of the pelvis (with its five fused vertebrae).

Many tai chi ch'uan movements originate in this particular region. These movements have a great influence on the form and function of the spinal column. This is one reason why people involved in tai chi ch'uan have no problems with scoliosis (bending of the spinal column to the side), or with kyphosis (bending backward), or with a "round back" (a condition that often occurs in the later years).

The gentle, flowing and arched movements involve many different muscles. However, there is no exertion and thereby they remain strong and limber and stay this way throughout life.

Muscles also have a strengthening effect on bone structure. The blood supply in the muscles and bones is stimulated through a better functioning digestive and metabolic system. Increased availability of calcium is achieved in particular.

Optimal conditioning of all joints, muscles, and ligaments is another advantage to be gained through tai chi ch'uan. Joints become stronger while their elasticity and flexibility is increased.

Meditation

Meditation is an attempt to be free of thoughts for a specific period of time in order to gain access to one's creative sources and riches. You will then be able to expand your consciousness, heighten your thought process, and increase your intuitive abilities. While meditation is mental emptiness, at the same time, it is in itself a mental process and shows a paradox. It is thus a good example of the Ying-Yang principle (of the philosophy of Taoism), the concept of passivity (Ying—mental emptiness) and activity (Yang—mental activity) to reach "emptiness."

The Ying and the Yang are in direct relationship to each other and at the same time opposites. For instance, in the Ying phase there is always a certain amount of Yang present: even in the most quiet and deepest moments during meditation (the Ying), one needs to pay attention (the Yang) to the breathing process in order to achieve the lowering of Qi into Dan-Tian. Yang also has an element of Ying present: one must have quiet and calm in order to concentrate on the above described process. If one of these principles were to be eliminated, life would cease to exist, according to Taoism.

Likewise, we cannot stop thinking, consciously or unconsciously, as long as we are alive. Thoughts are always present, and in order to achieve that moment during meditation where one is relatively free of rambling thoughts, one must first accept their existence. If you give them a place in your consciousness they will stop interfering, and most of the time will disappear on their own.

Tai chi ch'uan creates a good atmosphere for successful meditation through the intensive concentration on the movements and the process of lowering the Qi into the Dan-Tian. This concentration turns off the interferences from the inside as well as from the outside. The erect posture, gentle movements and proper breathing are also of great help to meditation.

The typical body posture (straight spine, knees slightly bent) may seem uncomfortable in the beginning but, after an initial period of getting used to, will allow the body to relax. When all muscles and joints are free of tension and when proper breathing has been accomplished, people who practise tai chi ch'uan will have a sense of well-being that is like a nectar for the soul. This state of mental and physical relaxation will create a state of total harmony.

Thus, tai chi ch'uan represents one of the best means for promoting mental calmness and the ability of looking within, of becoming one with oneself. To make it possible to reach this goal of meditation, one must create certain conditions, including a quiet place, fresh air, good light, and comfortable clothing.

Try to practise tai chi ch'uan as correctly as possible. Remember:

- correct posture
- gentle, round movements
- well-timed body coordination
- expressive display of positions
- flowing transition (shifting body weight and position)
- intentional display of movements
- proper breathing
- lowering Qi into Dan-Tian.

It should be remembered that one can only achieve a state of deep inner quietness when meditation itself is not an effort; this is true for any kind of meditation. The better the form is done, the easier it is to reach. People sometimes work for months (or even years) to achieve this inner peace. Remember, though, once the journey has begun every step will bring you closer to your goal, no matter how far away. The journey itself is the goal.

If you practise with patience and calmness you will be able to do the exercises with ever-increasing correctness, and your efforts will pay off. Even if highest perfection is almost impossible to obtain, you will get better with every exercise: better posture, better position of movements, a better breathing technique and an improvement in Qi.

Highest perfection seems
to be unattainable,
but its application is
unfailing.

Abundance seems to be empty
but its usefulness
is endless.

Greatest honesty seems
to be unscrupulous—
greatest skill seems
to be inept—
powerful rhetoric appears
to be ponderous.

Calmness will overcome chaos,
Coolness will overcome heat.
Peace and tranquility
are an example
for all of us.

(Tao-Te-Ching, chapter 45)

Individual positions will become more expressive through continued practice. The essence of tai chi ch'uan will begin to unfold after a certain mastery has been achieved, and then you can begin to experience, in a physical sense, the Ying-Yang principle and the centering of Qi into Dan-Tian. It is in this form that we can get a sense of the Ying-Yang principles:

- Burdening and unburdening
- Giving and taking
- Gentleness and strength
- Pulling back and stepping forward
- Giving and taking

The same holds true for the process of Qi into Dan-Tian: The attempt to center Qi, which is our total consciousness, into Dan-Tian, which is our body's center (center of the abdomen) is the same as searching for a mental and psychological balance.

In China it is often called: "The balance between Ying and Yang," or: "The harmony between body and soul." In essence it means the wholeness of the human being.

All this it not to imply that meditation asks us to turn our back on the world in which we live. Rather, meditation should give you the opportunity to find your Self so that you may be able to live consciously, and realize your essential humanness. The principles of Ying-Yang and the understanding of our own center which we learn through the practise of tai chi ch'uan are meant to help us live our everyday life. Only then can there be harmony between inner awareness (the Ying) and the outer world (the Yang). Through meditation Ying gains in strength and through practical application Yang becomes more secure. The harmony between Ying (inner knowledge) and Yang (care for the necessities of life) enable a human being to be whole. This is the essence of the philosophy of Taoism: the understanding of the true journey of the human being.

When body and soul
are in harmony with each other
how can you distinguish
one from the other?

When you have achieved inner peace
by yielding completely,
can you then act
like a newborn child?

When you have surrendered all confusing thoughts
and are clear within yourself,
can you say you have no flaws?

If you love your people
and are ready to serve your country,
can you be uninvolved?

If you are conscious
of your environment,
can you be indifferent?

If you love and trust
all things and your neighbor,
can you remain untouched?

(Tao-Te-Ching, Chapter 10)

Index